Carla Christy  No Accident

Advance Praise

"Carla Christy's book is a must read for anyone who is a family member of a head injury survivor. This well-written book by a mother of a brain injury survivor is truly an affirmation that there is hope for the victims of traumatic brain injury."

—Gary Jarvis, PhD. Clinical Neurophysiologist

"I was amazed and touched by her ability to capture in words the unbelievable array of conflicting emotions of fear, hope, sadness and devastation that most families experience. I hope this book will get into the hands of those who need it, when they need it most and help offer comfort and insight into the normalcy of these thoughts, questions, feelings of hopefulness and helplessness, faithfulness and loss of faith, sorrow and sometimes joy that accompany those who are suddenly thrust into the terrifying and unknown world of TBI".

—Kathy Martin, M.Ed, CRC, CPCRT, CBIST

"Carla Christy's hand is outstretched, proffering the gift of hope so desperately needed to those whose lives have been torn apart by traumatic brain injury. I hope that this book becomes part of every ICU, neurology & rehab unit's reading collection. It is an inspiration to patient, family members & medical caregiver alike. It is a reminder to me that every person's journey is unique and, one should never lose sight of that fact."

—Kathy Brady, CRNP

"No Accident is a deeply moving testament to the power of a mother's Love. Heartwarming, poignant; a message of what can be accomplished through acceptance, faith and determination."

—Lynn Bricker, C.O.T.A -L

"I have had the remarkable privilege of journeying with Carla and her son, Orion Christy, during the latter's rehabilitation. This family has experienced the depths of despair and, through their struggle, now have a remarkable story and gift to share with others. No Accident is an inspiring account of relentless perseverance and hope through the frightening journey of recovering from traumatic brain injury. It will surely be a great source of strength, insight, help and encouragement for families of those who have experienced traumatic brain injury."

—Suzanne Glaze, OTRL, CHT

"My life was over the day my wife sustained TBI in an accident. We had built a life of love together, but in an instant all that we had worked for was ripped away. I didn't think that I could go on. In my own dark night of the soul, I entertained the murky thoughts of a person who felt that life had become meaningless and pointless. But when I read Carla Christy's No Accident, I realized that she and her family had gone through the hell on earth that I had –and not only survived, but found a way to thrive. I didn't think that was possible. At many of the TBI and neurology-based support groups that I attended, I saw empty eyes and heard the raw, breaking hearts of those who believed that hope had abandoned them. People just like me. That changed when I read this book. I discovered through Carla's story, that not only can I find a reason to survive, but that I can build a new life beyond TBI. All that I can say is:

Read this book. Please don't wait. <u>There is hope</u>".

—Henry Trask, family member of a TBI victim

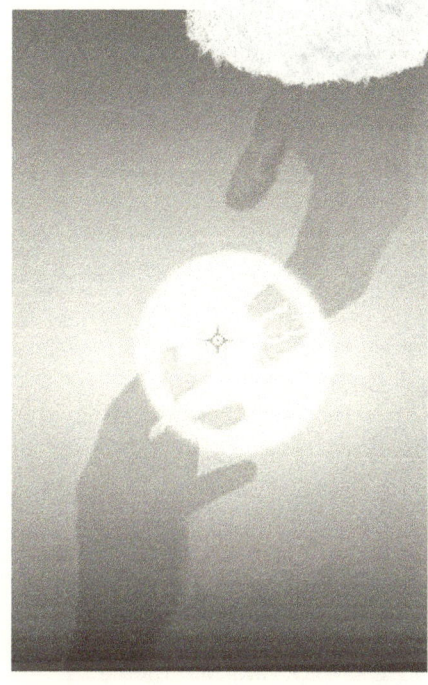

CARLA CHRISTY

MOTHER AND NURSE

Foreword by
**Charles Whitfield, MD
&
Barbara Harris Whitfield**

NO ACCIDENT

Hope for Victims of Traumatic Brain Injury and Their Families

*Finding the Inner Strength
To Handle Life's Challenges*

MHP
muse house press

Muse House Press

ISBN: 978-1-935827-12-2

Trade Paperback (*also available on Kindle*)
Copyright © 2012 Carla Faith Christy
All Rights Reserved

Visit us on the Internet at:
    NoAccidentCarla@blogspot.com
    NoAccidentCarla.com

Muse House Press and the MHP Logo are imprints of Muse House Press

Cover design, Interior composition and prepress by:
Donald Brennan for Muse House Press / YakRider Media

Up to 5% of each chapter may be reproduced as quotes provided attribution to the author is made. Other use may be made only with prior written permission of the publisher.

    Direct requests to: NoAccidentCarla@gmail.com

Beach and cover photographs courtesy of Sheila Burger, used by permission.

Printed in the United States of America

First printing

DEDICATION

-This book is dedicated to my sons,

To my beautiful son, Noah:
I want you to know how proud I am of your courage.
I feel as if I wasn't there enough for you during your brother's recovery.
I want you to know that you were with me in my heart every second of every day.

I never left you for a minute.
Son, thank you for being so brave and strong.
Always know how much I love you and how very proud of you I am.
You mean the world to me!

To my wonderful son, Orion:
Because of your inner strength and determination, you made it to where you are today.

I hope you know how much you mean to me and how proud of you I am.
I appreciate your words of encouragement that kept me going when doubt tried to creep in. "Never give up Mom - ever!"
I love you, son!

FOREWORD

Charles L Whitfield, MD
Barbara H Whitfield, RT

This book does exactly what the title promises and more.

As a physician and respiratory therapist, we both have experienced *watching* the care and rehabilitation of catastrophically brain injured patients (Traumatic Brain Injury or TBI). It is a painfully slow process with an unknown outcome. And at the same time we have witnessed the significant others of these patients slowly crumble over the patient's and their own current helplessness and pain compounded by the clinical staff's inability to predict what is and what will happen.

The brain is an awesome organ. As sophisticated as modern medicine is, the part we know the least about is our human brain. It is the most puzzling and mysterious part of our human anatomy. Many theories about the brain are still only theories. As an example, this claim of serotonin in the brain (or lack of it) causing "depression" has never been proven in scientific research.

If we took everything we know about the brain and added it up --- it would not begin to equal what we don't know about it.

So in nearly all the cases of Traumatic Brain Injury there are no predictors. Waiting patiently is the only way to know what will happen. In this book, the author and definitely "heroine" Carla Christy shares with us her painful task of patiently sitting by her son Orion's bedside, praying, hoping, willing him to make a recovery that his first health care team had predicted would never happen. *She never stopped believing* that some day he would become a whole and independent human being. She takes us inside her heart and shows us her process of "believing him to recover."

She writes:

"It was a mother's intuition, something no words could ever fully describe. I believe intuition to be divine guidance; the God within talking to us on a deeper level. Our intuition is God's way of guiding us to the right path. It's that inner knowledge or gut feeling that will always guide us to the right path if we learn to trust it".

Carla gracefully shows us how being the caregiver in such a catastrophic injury is possible by explaining how she used her heart/intuition to guide her. Of course, her training as a nurse helps too. But nursing is taught mainly about science and Carla's strength comes in her *art* of nursing, intuition and love. She even shows us that she loves herself enough to take all the help that is offered to her by her family and friends so she avoids suffering "burn out." (This happens often in caregivers because they forget or don't know how important it is to take care of themselves.)

The journey in this book happens from the moment the author hears the terrible news of her son Orion's accident, through his first critical days, then through the endless months of rehabilitation. And at all times she keeps this vision of her son:

"Orion stood before [us] as a living example that anything is possible. The theme of his story encouraged [us] to never give up."

In the end, willingly, she steps aside and watches her son bond with others and eventually move out on his own. This perhaps, is one of the most important steps in recovery from catastrophic illness or injury for the caregiver – to be able to let go, step aside and start the ominous job of once again creating a new life because their old one ended when the catastrophe began.

In January, 2011, while attending a Co-Dependence Anonymous

Retreat in Hilton Head Island where I, Barbara was invited to teach, I walked with 10 or 11 women I had never met to a restaurant near the hotel for lunch. It is "No Accident" that I sat opposite Carla Christy and in the way that strangers often start a conversation, Carla mentioned that she was a nurse. So I told her I was a respiratory therapist. She went on to tell me that she had just finished caring for her son who had a Traumatic Brain Injury. Having worked with TBIs, I became interested and invited her to tell me the story.

With tears in my eyes, being able to feel what Carla was feeling because of her excellent ability to explain on a heart level, I said, "Carla, you ought to write this all in a book. You can help so many that will have to endure what you have been through."

So what you the reader hold in your hands right now is the gift of Carla's wisdom, steadfastness and "art of her nursing heart."

We are glad you found this book and it is probably no accident that you did. We wish you the best on your journey to help yourself and/or another recover from any kind of catastrophic illness or injury.

Charles L Whitfield, MD
Barbara H Whitfield, RT
Atlanta Georgia

The Whitfields are best-selling authors of **Healing the Child Within**, **Victim to Survivor Then Thriver,** and **Wisdom to Know the Difference: Core Issues in Relationships, Recovery and Living** (Learn more at the Resources section of this book.)

Barbara-Whitfield.blogspot.com

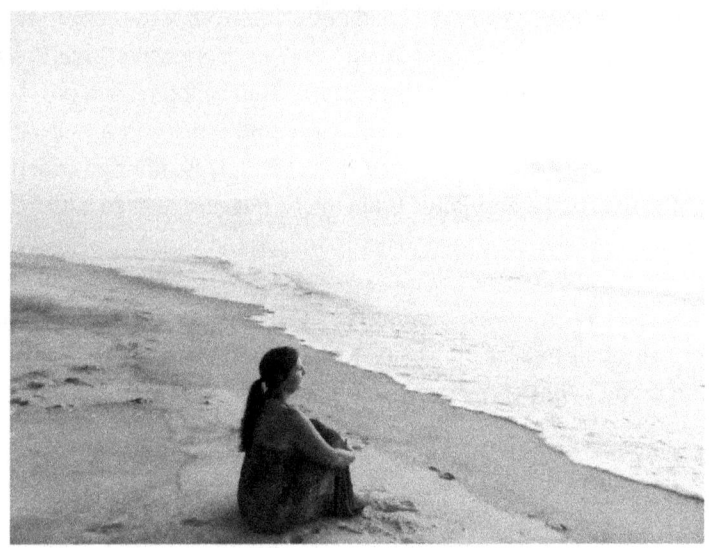

PREFACE

One day while sitting outside the therapy room, my mind raced with so many questions for God. Why my son? Why him, God? I was angry, frightened and confused so I picked up a pen and paper and started writing.

God, why my son? As I began to write the answers would come. I could feel the bottled up emotions pouring onto the paper while tears rolled down my cheeks. Several weeks later as my son began to recover, moments of joy crept onto the pages.

The early stages of his recovery reminded me of a newborn baby as it develops from infancy. Only my baby boy was six feet tall and 175 pounds! His journey back to adulthood would be a difficult one. Orion would re-learn to dress and feed himself, walk, talk, and polish the many social skill sets that develop along the way. My son's ultimate goal was to drive again, while ours was for him to regain total independence.

My husband and I wish to extend our gratitude and love for all the family, friends and loved ones who stood by our side. Our son's recovery would not have been possible without each and every one of you and your support. Each of you, like a thread in a tapestry, played a vital part in our son's recovery, and for that we will be forever grateful.

ACKNOWLEDGMENTS

I would like to extend my deepest gratitude to all my friends and family that were there for me during my son's recovery. You all mean the world to me!

To my eldest son Orion for your inspiration, to my precious son Noah for your strength and love, to my loving husband Bill for standing by our side.

To my parents, Rene and Ray, who I admire and who are the foundation of which I find my strength, my little sister Rhonda, her husband Dale and their children for whom I cherish, my older sister Debbie, her husband Bill and their children who I love with all my heart, and to my sister that I love and miss and whom I will never forget, Monica.

Pop for your unconditional love and GeGe for always guiding me in the right direction and watching over us each and every day. Becky and Bill for taking us into their home, your support and love mean the world to me and Robin and Dee for all the cards and prayers.

To my closest friends and spiritual sisters, Vicki for being such a special friend and someone I can always count on, Suzie for your love, encouragement and friendship, Helen for believing in miracles and believing in me and Deb and John for your prayers love and support. To my dear friend Sheila, without her, this book would never have happened; I can never tell you how much I appreciate all that you did to help me get this book out there. To Val for my holy water and to Linda and her beautiful daughter, Christine, for visiting so often. Your presence made such a difference and was so appreciated.

To my spiritual sisters Betty for holding Orion in the light, Logan for being the light being that you are, Kris, Cheryl, Nancy for your love and light and support. To the Buddhist monk, Michael, who will always have a special place in my heart.

To Tom and Andrea for being such good friends to Bill and I and for your love and support.

Thank you to all Orion's faithful friends that never gave up on him: Kelly, JT, Joey, Dante, Tarik, Jon, Justin, Lee, Rob and Ty and to Mr. Brazell for being a role model and for the encouragement you gave Orion and for most of all believing in him.

Thank you to all Noah's friends, especially Hunter and Lance, and their mothers, who took Noah under their wings when I couldn't be there.

Our entire family wishes to extend our deepest gratitude to all the therapists, doctors and nurses for you hard work and dedication.

To my publisher Donald Brennan for believing in my book and encouraging me along the way, my editor Lisa Keller for your input and advice, and to Charles and Barbara Whitfield for support and belief in my message.

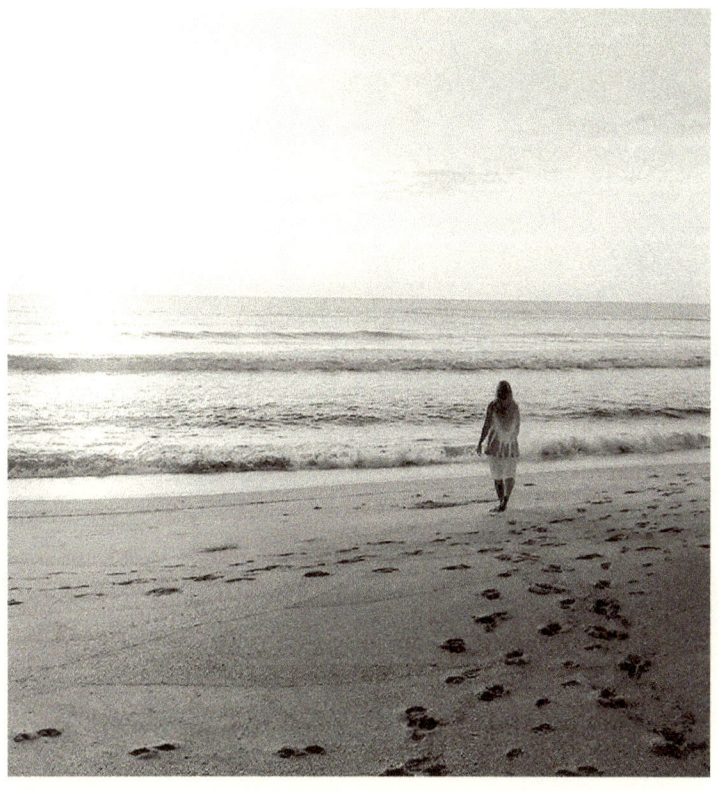

INTRODUCTION

It all started when I was a young girl in my mid twenties. I married straight out of high school and, needless to say, it didn't even last a year. I welcomed the move to Florida with my mom and little sister and settled in the small town of Flagler Beach. I was an independent, young waitress living in a small trailer and barely making enough money to pay the rent and other bills. Despite the struggle, I was very happy to leave the cold Kentucky weather and memories of the failed marriage.

I loved everything about Florida; the beaches, sun and ocean breezes. I especially loved the ocean. I was never afraid of the water and swimming in the ocean made me feel complete. The sound of the waves crashing against the shoreline, the ocean breeze, and of course, the feel of the refreshing water made me feel alive. I could swim for hours, but what really made my day was taking the time to lie in the sun and feel its warmth on my face. This was a rare occasion since I had rent to pay, yet somehow I always managed to get by.

One day I decided to watch the local surfers. They made it look so easy! I always wanted to learn to surf but I never had the guts. I chose to stick with swimming, but deep inside, I had an urge to someday give it a try. At that moment, I just watched in amazement.

There was one particular surfer that caught my eye. He always seemed to be in the right spot at the right time and made riding the waves look so effortless. I watched for hours as the day drifted away. Later I noticed the surfer as he got out of the water. In short, he was gorgeous! The thought left as quickly as it came as I turned and walked away. I wasn't interested in getting involved in a relationship at this point in my life.

Several weeks later I was out with my sister at a local establishment. The same surfer guy I had admired weeks before approached my sister and began talking to her. When I asked my sister what he said, she replied, "He wanted to know all about you." "Really," I asked her, pleasantly surprised. Later that evening he finally got the nerve to ask me out on our first date.

When he came to pick me up I had a steak cooking on the grill. Later that evening we were skating at the boardwalk and talking about surfing, beaches and health. I was embarrassed to learn he didn't eat meat. After that night, I too became a vegetarian and also found my soul mate. We had a lot in common, but most importantly, Bill and I had fallen in love at first sight.

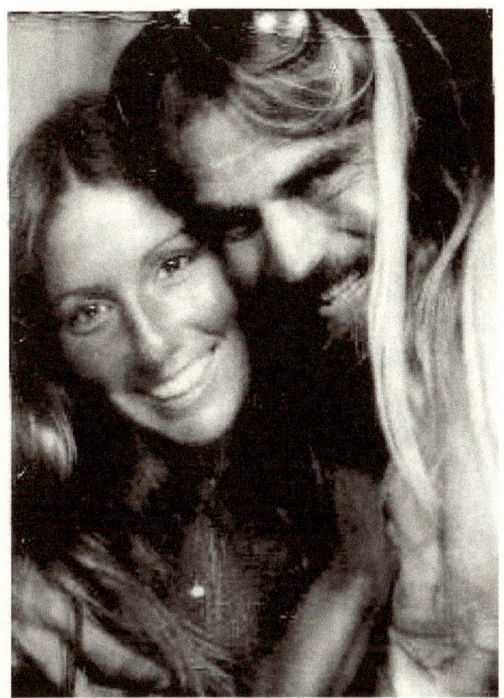

Bill and Carla: on our first date at the boardwalk

We moved into our first home. It was an old boat with, shall we say 'lots of character,' including a hole in the bottom. But it was our beginning, and it was beautiful. I started nursing school. Bill was a carpenter by trade and worked at a local boat factory. Our life was wonderful and we were very much in love.

I became pregnant with our first son in 1984. His name was originally to be Jordon. One evening before his birth we gazed together at the constellation Orion in the night sky. When our son was born he was large and strong like the hunter Orion. So his name became Orion Jordon.

We raised our son in our second home which was a sailboat. Orion loved living on the boat. His bedroom was the bow with a few toys lining his bunk. He didn't need much to be happy. The sound of the waves splashing on the side of the boat seemed to bring a feeling of comfort and tranquility to our young son. The crystals hanging from the windows amazed him and the flickering of their rainbow in the cabin entertained him for hours. He enjoyed the warmth of the sun and the salt life lifestyle from a young age.

Orion was a natural on the deck as he moved effortlessly around the cabin like nothing was impossible. In fact he learned at a very early age to pull himself up and walk around the vessel within the boundaries of the netting we had installed to ensure his safety. We used to laugh because on land, it was quite a different story. He would sway on land like most people would sway on a boat at sea.

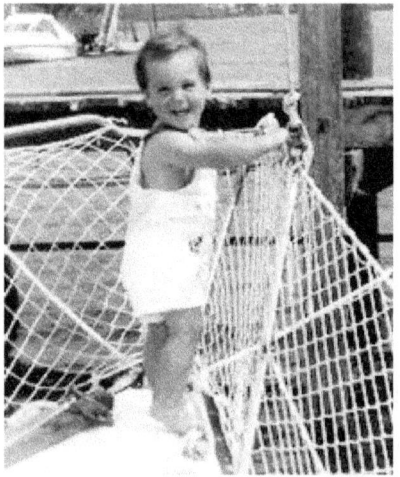

Orion on the bow of the boat

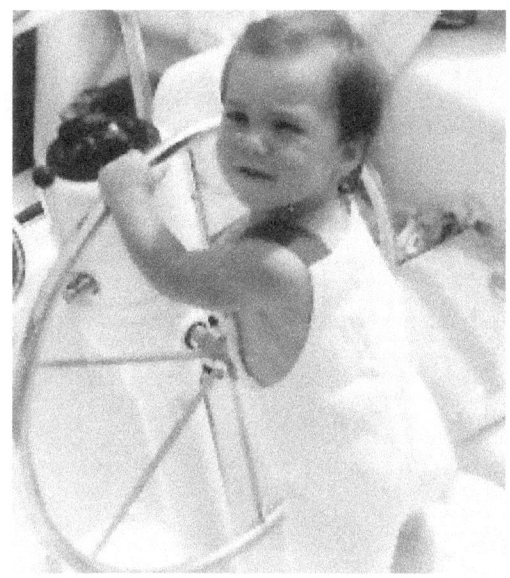

Orion at the helm

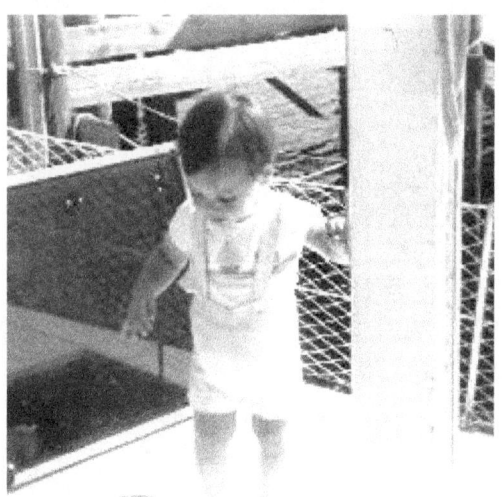

Orion getting around on the boat

Our son had an operation at an early age to address a cataract that he had since birth. Afterwards he had to wear a patch over one eye while the other eye healed. But that didn't seem to slow down our determined young son. He wore the patch proudly and fit in even better at the marina with the other sea faring residents.

Living on the boat was wonderful and the memories live on in my heart to this day. I recall the sparkling light dancing on the water, the sunbaths on the deck, the occasional passing by of a manatee and her calf and those beautiful starlit nights as if it were yesterday.

Three and a half years later we were thrilled to expect our second child and were blessed with a beautiful baby boy. He was a happy, easy going baby who came into this world smiling and good natured. There was never a doubt that God had blessed us with our beach baby. So we called him Noah Sea. We felt as though God had given us one baby from the heavens and one baby from the sea.

Noah was such a precious sweet child, a true gift from God. His eyes were blue and he had fine, curly blond hair. His smile was so sweet and innocent. Noah seemed amazed at the world and everything in it. When I took him near the ocean it was like he became one with it. I could see at a very early age his bright eyes twinkled and his face lit up each time when he heard the word 'beach'.

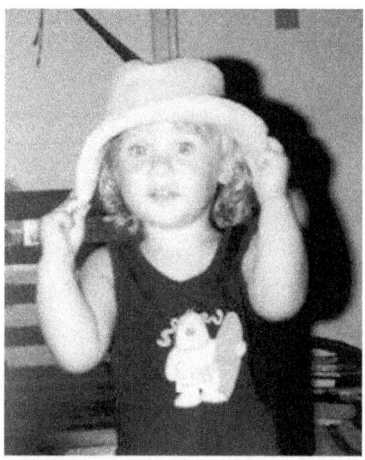
Noah, my blue-eyed surfer boy

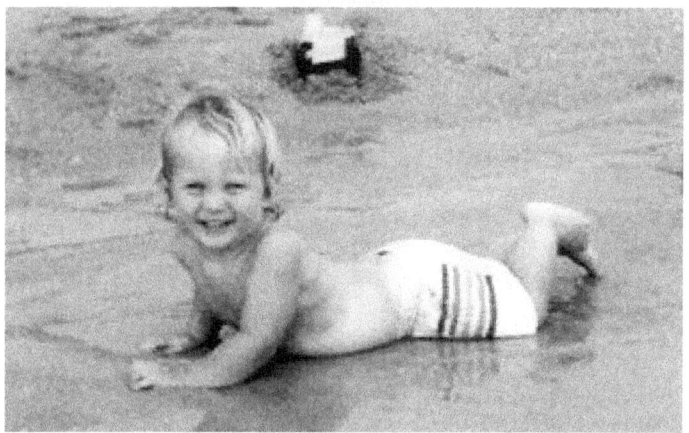
Noah at the beach

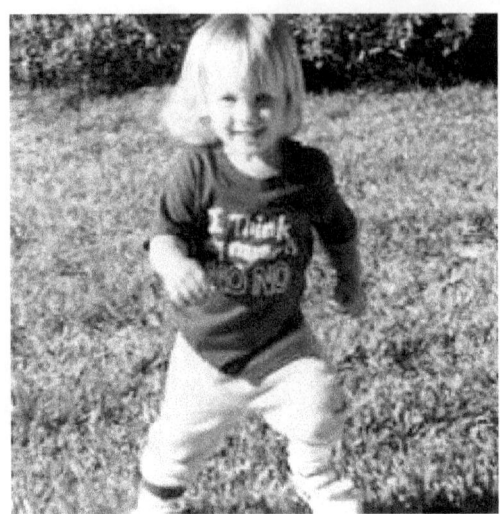

Noah in action

With the arrival of our new son we decided to rent a 2 bedroom apartment. I wasn't quite certain I could handle two young boys on the boat and this way they could have their own room. I remember when my husband and I first arrived at the apartment and opened the door. I said, "Wow look how big it is!" I think at that very moment Bill and I knew the days of living on a boat were over.

We loved our boys and there was nothing as important to us as the two of them. As the years rolled by and the boys grew we enjoyed all the stages of their lives. They were involved in baseball, soccer, surfing, boy scouts, skateboarding and even karate.

The years passed so quickly, and as my story begins, my precious young boys are seventeen and twenty years old. Noah was enjoying his final year of high school and spending most of his time with his friends at the beach. He loved the ocean, and surfing had become Noah's passion. It is a love inherited from his father.

Orion had moved to Orlando, attended film school and graduated. He was a self-motivated, good student and enjoyed his privacy. He had moved back home nearly two weeks prior to his twenty-first birthday to save money and gather his belongings. His ultimate plan was to relocate to California with his friends and pursue a career in film. Orion's passion surrounded the movie industry and a career in film was his dream.

On April 2, 2006 our lives were turned upside down. This book is a story of survivorship and hope. It describes my journey and how I somehow found the inner strength to face life's challenges. My wish is that this story will help my readers discover their inner strength as they make their way through their own difficult situations. Never give up!

THE ACCIDENT

It was 4:30 a.m. and we were awakened by a knock on the door. I could hear my husband talking in a trembling voice but couldn't make out what the other person was saying. I got out of bed and looked out the window to see a police car driving away. My whole body was shaking. I knew something had happened. Before I could get up and make it downstairs, my young son, Noah, stood at the end of my bed, his eyes filled with tears. My husband's voice quivered as he said, "There's been an accident and we need to get to the hospital." The police officer had handed my husband a piece of paper and told him that Orion, our twenty year old son, had been in a terrible car accident and was in critical condition at a hospital in a nearby town.

His voice still trembling, Bill took my hand and said, "Come on. Let's get going." Noah, just seventeen years old, stood in our room shaking, with the look of worry in his beautiful blue eyes. I held Noah tightly and reassured him that everything was going to be alright. Actually, I was in shock. My hands shook uncontrollably as I read the paper the officer had handed my husband. It stated Orion was in critical condition, that his car had gone into the intra coastal waterway and was a possible drowning and/or spinal cord injury. The word "critical" stood out on the paper. At this point, my nursing background only made matters worse. I knew if he had gone under water he may not survive.

The ride to the hospital was horrific. Tears poured down my husband's face as he drove. I felt as if my insides were dying; my nerves were shot and I was in complete panic mode because I had no idea if Orion was going to be alive. I wondered where and how this happened, but most importantly, why our son? It was a forty minute drive to the hospital, but it seemed as though it took hours. All I wanted was to get to my eldest son's side.

When we finally arrived at the hospital, we were told Orion had undergone brain surgery. Part of his skull had been removed so the surgeons could operate. He had a major hemorrhage, a 2.3 cm. bleed in his brain. His prognosis was grim. He had suffered a very severe Traumatic Brain Injury (TBI) and was a 3 on the Glasgow coma scale.

In terms of head injuries, doctors often use numbers on a scale of 1-15 to describe the level of injury. A fifteen means there is no mental injury or impairment noted. Seven usually means the patient is comatose and three indicates probable brain death. One or two means the patient is either dead or death is imminent. In Orion's case, the value of three meant that *if* he survived, he would most likely be very severely brain damaged. In addition, they were not yet sure whether or not he had suffered a spinal cord injury. He was in the intensive surgical care unit on life support.

The document on the following page offers detail as to how the Glasgow numbers are derived.

FACTS: THE SEVERITY OF BRAIN INJURY

Emergency personnel typically determine the severity of a brain injury by using an assessment called the Glasgow Coma Scale (GCS). The terms Mild Brain Injury, Moderate Brain Injury, and Severe Brain Injury are used to describe the level of initial injury in relation to the neurological severity caused to the brain. ***There may be no correlation between the initial Glasgow Coma Scale score and the initial level of brain injury and a person's short or long term recovery, or functional abilities.*** Keep in mind that there is nothing "Mild" about a brain injury—the term "Mild" Brain injury is used to describe a level of neurological injury. Any injury to the brain is a real and serious medical condition. There is additional information about mild brain injury on our mild brain injury page.

Glasgow Coma Score (GCS)		
Eye Opening (E)	Verbal Response (V)	Motor Response (M)
4=Spontaneous	5=Normal conversation	6=Normal
3=To voice	4=Disoriented conversation	5=Localizes to pain
2=To pain	3=Words, but not coherent	4=Withdraws to pain
1=None	2=No words .only sounds	3=Decorticate posture
	1=None	2=Decerebrate
		1=None
		Total = E+V+M

The scale comprises three tests: eye, verbal and motor responses. The three values separately as well as their sum are considered. The lowest possible GCS (the sum) is 3 (deep coma or death), while the highest is 15 (fully awake person). A GCS score of 13-15 is considered a "mild" injury; a score of 9-12 is considered a moderate injury; and 8 or below is considered a severe brain injury.

From Brain Injury Association of America. (2012). In *About Brain Injury*, find *Severity of Brain Injury*. Retrieved June 13, 2012.

www.biausa.org/Default.aspx?PageID=3597010&A=SearchResult&SearchID=4388867&ObjectID=3597010&ObjectType=1#definitions

The nurse met us as we approached his room. She explained that Orion was in critical condition and they were unsure if he would survive the night. Orion was on a ventilator and his heart rate was in the 180's. His condition was comatose and there were tubes everywhere, including those coming out of his head. The bone flap of his skull had been removed and half his head was shaved. I heard words like questionable drowning, craniotomy, decerebrate posturing, pneumothorax, fractured ribs and massive hemorrhage of the brain. Although my nursing background had exposed me to medical terms such as these, nothing was registering in my mind.

This was *my* child lying there and I was overwhelmed with emotion. Meanwhile, my youngest son Noah stood solemnly looking at his brother. I prayed as we cried and stared at Orion's motionless body. I felt very helpless as my son lay there, heart rate tacking and blood pressure dropping. I could not do this!

Throughout the night we felt increasingly helpless. Worst of all was that we did not know if he would wake up. *If* he did awake, would he even know who we were, or would he be the 'vegetable' the doctors and nurses spoke of over and over? So many emotions ran through our minds. I had never been so frightened in my life. Noah and I held each other as my husband tried to comfort us both. I tried to reassure Noah that his brother would be alright, but deep inside anxiety and fear raged on. Over and over I pleaded with God to please let my son live.

I was so very grateful Orion had made it through the first night. My mother and sister arrived that morning and I noticed my sister talking to the neurosurgeon. The looks on their faces were not promising. She later told me that the doctor had said, "It is really bad and we are just not sure if he is going to survive." His prognosis was still grim.

The hallways were lined with many of Orion's friends that came to see him. Unfortunately, his condition was too critical to have visitors outside the immediate family. They were disappointed that they were not permitted in the room, but understood the rule was in place to protect Orion. That didn't stop them from dropping by the hospital regularly to check on his condition. I was so pleased to see such support and heartfelt concern from so many.

Much to my surprise, later that day I shared the elevator with a young, Asian girl. She stood beside me crying, so I asked her if she was okay. She told me that her boyfriend had been in an accident. Tears welled up in my eyes as I said, "Honey I'm sorry, my son was also in an accident." She went on to tell me that her name was Ada and her boyfriend's name was Orion. I was shocked. We were unaware of Orion's new friend. We hugged for a moment and then I was called by the nurse to return to the station.
--
Hours turned into days and days into weeks as we sat by Orion's side hoping and praying that he would wake up. As if his condition was not bad enough, Orion developed an infection from the canal water

he had swallowed prior to his rescue. The infection caused his temperature to rise so the nurses wrapped him in a cooling blanket which made his body shake violently. It was so hard to watch our child, someone we loved with all our hearts, freezing and shaking, barely hanging on. I wanted to wrap him in my arms as I did when he was a baby and hold and comfort him.

Day in and day out Orion lay listless with the exception of his violently shaking body. The nurses would pinch him to try and get a response but there was no reaction. I spent long days at his bedside pleading to God to please bring our son back to us. Depending on the nurses and hospital staff, I could sometimes sit with him for hours and other times in fifteen minute intervals.

When I couldn't be by his side, I would sit in a rose garden just outside the hospital where I pleaded, begged and prayed. I had so many questions for God. How could this be happening? Why my son? Was it something I did? Or something I didn't do? My prayers in the rose garden brought a calmness and peace I didn't know was possible during such a traumatic time. There was something very precious about that place. Unfortunately the anxiety and fear quickly returned the second I left my temporary sanctuary.

One day at the hospital I was trembling and my little sister, Ronnie had wrapped a small purple sheet around my arms. That little sheet brought me such comfort. I would bring it with me and sit on it in the rose garden while I connected to God. My mom, little sister and Bill would come to check on me, but they understood I had to be alone in my rose garden talking to God. My sister Debbie called my mom daily to check on Orion and me. I loved her so much and knew she was just a phone call away and that was also comforting to me. I felt so blessed to have such a loving family.

My life remained focused solely on Orion. I made my way through most days on very little sleep. Food was repulsive and my mind foggy. I wandered around in a daze. All I knew to do was pray. Nothing in this world is as important to me as my boys. They are my life. The thought of losing either of them was more than I could comprehend.

Faith was my middle name and I decided my mom had given it to me for a reason. It was time to turn to that faith. In the scripture, it reads 'All things I do you too can do.' My spiritual practice had taught me to decree a thing and it shall be. So my daily mantra became, 'I am the resurrection and life of Orion's perfectly healed mind, body and spirit.' In addition, each time I entered the hospital and passed by the huge statue of big gold hands, I pictured them as God's hands holding my son's brain and healing him.

Sometimes I went to the hospital chapel. Each visit I was on my knees begging God to bring my son back to me. As Easter grew near, I placed a flower beside a picture of Orion that remained in the chapel.

I thought this to be a time of resurrection and I wanted so much for my son to resurrect, just as God's Son had done. I prayed, "Please God. Please bring our son back to us."

Easter came and went. Orion turned twenty-one years old a week later. It had been over two weeks since the accident. He spent his birthday comatose in a hospital bed. I thought this isn't the way it's supposed to be when you turn twenty-one. There should be parties and celebrations, not this! I was overcome with sadness, but I never gave up. It was a bittersweet time, sad and angry about the accident yet grateful my son was still with us.

The days seemed endless as I sat helplessly by my son's side. The nights were even worse. I couldn't be with him, but neither would I leave the hospital. When I finally slept it was from pure exhaustion. I would awaken throughout the night very disoriented and not knowing what had happened. I'd panic and think it was all a bad dream. Then I remembered this nightmare was real. The tears streamed down my cheeks as I cried and cried and couldn't seem to stop. I attempted to calm myself and breathe. My husband would try to calm me. But the tears flowed endlessly. I just wanted morning to come so I could be back by Orion's side.

I hardly saw Noah as I spent my time at the hospital with Orion. My husband and I had decided to expose Noah to his brother's condition as little as possible. We tried to believe he was living a 'normal' life, but the reality was our younger son was struggling too. He relied on his friends to help him through his days. Noah tried to concentrate on his last year of high school but I could see the sadness and fear in his beautiful eyes. He was so young and innocent. When we did spend time together I didn't know what to say to help him. All I could do was hold him, cry with him and reassure him that his brother was going to be okay. The truth was that inside I was like a scared little girl myself.

FATE

Orion's car had been towed from the scene of the accident and our bill from the towing company was increasing with each additional day. It was time to go pay the towing company and collect our son's belongings. My husband tried to convince me not to go, but I knew in my heart I had to see the car for myself and begin to find closure.

First we visited the spot where the accident had occurred. It was a winding back road lined with palm and old oak trees along the waterways. I was told that my son was traveling at the posted speed limit of 25 M.P.H. when most likely an animal had run across his path. The officers had noted they encountered many deer on their way to the scene of the accident that night. They determined he had swerved to miss an animal, slammed sideways into a palm tree on the edge of the canal and lost control of the vehicle. His car struck the tree on the driver's side door where Orion took the full impact of the collision to his left side and head. The vehicle then plunged into the waterway at approximately 10:30 p.m. on a road traveled by very few people.

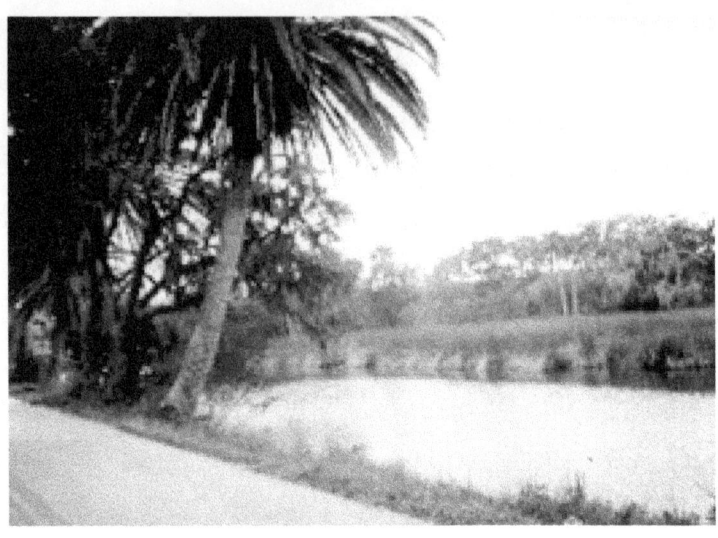

Photo of the accident location taken by Orion Christy

We later found out that one of Orion's school mates was headed home that evening when he saw headlights eerily shining in the water and phoned his mother who instructed him to call 911 for help. It was over a year before we knew who made the call that saved our son's life. We are so grateful he took action rather than simply passed by.

We drove to the towing company location. When we entered the tow yard we saw all the wrecked cars behind a gated area. As we approached Orion's car the sight of the crushed wreckage took my breath away. The driver's side of the car that had hit the tree was severely caved in. All of the glass was shattered and the steel bent beyond recognition. My heart sank. It was a very difficult experience, and the vision of his demolished car is a picture I will never forget.

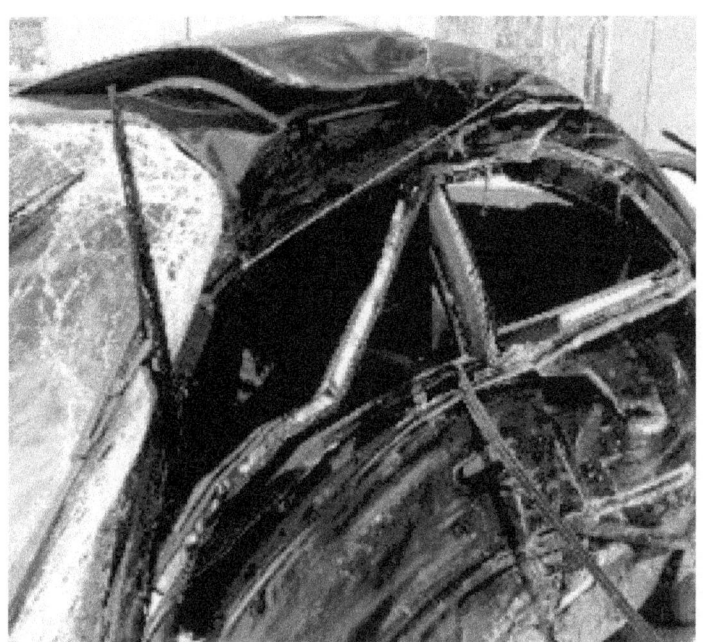

Photo of the mangled wreckage

Bill began to gather Orion's belongings and found his wallet on the dash. This explained why our son had been admitted to the hospital as a 'John Doe' and why so many hours had passed before we received the knock at our door. Everything had been buried deep in mud from the canal and the medics were unable to find any identification.

The police had summoned for a dive team to rescue my son from inside his car in the middle of the waterway. They also searched for possible passengers since he could not communicate that he was alone at the time of the accident. Because Orion's condition was critical, the paramedics had immediately airlifted him to the closest trauma unit. Afterward, they used the tag number on the license plate of his car to identify him and subsequently contact us at our home.

In the trunk were clothes, folders and lots of papers, all unrecognizable as they were covered with mud and still wet. My husband carefully collected everything and we continued on our way. I was glad I went with him but also glad the trip was over.

When we arrived back home, Bill spread out nearly a hundred papers he had found hoping to preserve anything possible. A few days later the papers were dry. All of them were smudged and unreadable except one which appeared to be untouched. It contained a few lines written by our son. As I read the words, my eyes filled with tears but my heart was full of hope. Over and over again I repeated to myself, 'With God, all things are possible.' I felt this was a message from God. Orion had entitled the paper FATE. Here are his words:

FATE

If our destiny is in fact pre-determined then it must remain hidden in order to preserve the struggle. This is not intended to make life difficult but to keep it interesting and meaningful, a journey's end that is revealed before the start is not one worth undertaking. Adventure is in our very beings, it helps drive us, and keeps us entertained. The frustration that overwhelms is due to unacceptance of the truth, a destructive state that only further clouds life's mysteries. Surely all of mine are speculation but I believe this too to be an adventure in enlightenment.

Orion Christy

MIRACLES

I believe our faith is challenged throughout our lifetime for reasons most of us cannot begin to understand. During such times we pray for God's miraculous love to bring peace to our soul. We ask Him to walk by our side and give us strength and courage to overcome whatever obstacle has darkened our perfectly lit pathway.

It was 'no accident' that my husband found Orion's amazingly preserved message to us among the many other ruined pages from the wreckage. His words gave us strength at a time when our hearts were saddened beyond belief and our faith was at an all time low. How could we know that our critically injured son would communicate his inspirational message to us and reaffirm our faith in God's miraculous power? As my story continues, my husband and I repeat our mantra, 'With God, all things *are* possible!' as we witness His miracles unfold.

Day in and day out we talked to Orion, held his hand and asked him to squeeze or open his eyes, hoping to get a response. Unfortunately, nothing happened as he lay there motionless. One morning the nurse told us the night nurse had seen Orion's eyes open for the first time since he was admitted. The news filled our hearts with joy and excitement. Sadly, when we asked him to open his eyes there was no response. The next day another nurse said she had a response when she asked him to squeeze her finger. But when we made the same request, again nothing happened. We were so grateful to receive good news yet frustrated when we could not see it for ourselves. Once again we turned to our faith. We had to 'let go and let God.' We knew it was all up to Him and we surrendered to that fact.

After approximately two and a half weeks in a coma, Orion started to open his eyes. He was unable to focus, yet I somehow knew he recognized my voice because he would flail his right side when I spoke to him as his left side remained paralyzed. Finally, a step forward! The weeks since the accident seemed like months while we waited for the slightest sign of improvement. And here it was. God had begun to answer our prayers and reveal His miraculous power.

Orion wasn't out of the woods yet. At this point, our son had undergone three more surgeries to drain the fluid that continuously collected around his brain. Bill and I made the tough decision to have a VP shunt surgically placed in his head to allow the fluid to drain rather than Orion enduring ongoing surgeries. The decision was difficult because once the shunt was inserted it would be with him the rest of his life. In addition, there was a feeding tube in his stomach and the doctors still had not replaced part of his skull, which would require yet another trip to the O.R.

The doctors also performed a tracheotomy which replaced the oral airway so Orion's mouth was clear. Afterward his teeth gritted so tight they had to use a bite block so he didn't bite his tongue. As the nurses tried to clean his mouth, crusty from weeks on the ventilator tube, Orion's teeth clinched tighter. I wondered if he knew what had happened, where he was or what the nurses were doing. Although his eyes were open, he was not able to communicate with us. There was simply a blank stare.

It was weeks in the Intensive Care Unit (ICU) before the doctors decided Orion was stable enough to transfer to a less critical setting. Finally, he was moved out of ICU into another room. God continued to answer our prayers. We were so grateful to move past the uncertainty that surrounded the ICU. Our son was alive and had moved into the recovery phase of his long journey back to us. I could feel God's presence and was thankful for this miraculous day.

Orion's left side still had no movement, but the rest of his body was extremely active. The nurses quickly realized he would require twenty-four hour supervision so he would not pull out all of the tubes. This was affirmed one night when the sitter had looked away for just a moment. Even though Orion's right hand was tied, he'd managed to rip out his *trache* tube which was his airway. The team ran frantically down the hall to his rescue. Thankfully, they were able to replace it without him going into respiratory distress. I wondered if he was frustrated or scared. What must he be thinking about during all of this? I prayed and asked God to bring comfort and peace to my son as he made his way back to us.

Since Orion had moved from ICU, it was time to determine the extent of damage to his motor skills. A physical therapist came to evaluate Orion's case. I watched the therapist attempt some range of motion exercises on my son. His body was like a limp wash rag. It would just fall to the side because he couldn't hold himself up. My heart broke and my insides felt as though they had crumbled apart. I tried to keep a smile as I spoke encouraging words to reassure Orion he was going to be just fine.

God sent one miracle after another during this stage of Orion's recovery. For example, Noah came to visit one day and I could see Orion light up. His body was weak but he recognized his brother. I knew this because although I was not sure if Orion could see his brother's precious eyes filling with tears, he seemed to be responding to Noah's voice. Most of the time he would just stare off into space but this day was different. Orion was trying to track his brother's voice with his eyes. It was an amazing site! Not only was he trying to focus his eyes, he was trying to hold his head up! I breathed a huge sigh of relief and my heart filled with joy. No longer did I question whether or not my son would recognize his family.

A few weeks later, Orion started trying to communicate. Initially, he used a thumb up for 'yes' and a thumb down for 'no'. As time passed, he graduated to using a letter or alphabet board. He would point so fast at each letter that there was no way to keep up without writing it down. At one point, he spelled out, 'I have a lot to say.' And I replied,

"I bet you do, son. And you will be able to. Just hang in there." We were having a conversation! My heart was full of anticipation and renewed hope. I wanted to hear everything he had to say!

I cherished such moments and was grateful as I witnessed God's miraculous power. Orion was making tremendous progress and each step forward was a blessing. I felt strength that I hadn't felt since before that fateful day. It was an inner knowledge that somehow, someway, my son was going to be okay.

I remember another day when Orion was lying there, leaning to his side, looking 'out of it.' That is until Noah walked in the room. His brother's presence caused him to light up like a Christmas tree! Once again Orion raised his head, eyes scanning the room to connect with his brother's voice. He had been left handed prior to the accident and now his hand lay lifeless on his lap with a squeeze ball inside to keep it open. Suddenly, he rolled the ball to his right hand and tossed it. I was shocked! Although his left side was still flaccid and most times he could barely hold his head up, Orion somehow managed to move that ball to his other hand and toss it to his brother. We were stunned! Noah looked at his brother, reached down, picked up the ball and tossed it back at him. Before I knew it they were tossing the ball back and forth to one another. Tears streamed down my cheeks, but this time they were tears of joy! That day I will treasure always. It's a day I will never forget. Pop and Bill were there too. I remember looking at their faces and saw smiles and heard laughter. We gave thanks to

God for answering our prayers. This was yet another sign that our son was coming back to us!

We cherished such glorious moments and used them to renew and strengthen our faith. As other people spoke of their TBI experiences, they insinuated Orion might never walk. Not in our world! They said he wouldn't talk either, but low and behold, he was getting close. Both Bill and I were determined not to give in to their negative beliefs. We held onto our mantra, 'With God, all things are possible.' We knew God had a plan for this brilliant, young man and they didn't know *our son*! We had already begun to see His miracles happening and clung onto the thought of *when* our son would walk, not *if* he would walk.

There had been moments of glory, excitement and joy among the many filled with frustration, fear and sadness. Regardless, my husband and I were blessed and grateful to witness several of God's miracles. The most important was He had restored life to our son's broken body.

RECOVERY

Our journey back had only just begun. The recovery process was long with many 'ups and downs.' There were moments when my fears surfaced, as well as those that warmed my heart and renewed my faith. As I accompanied my son on his long, difficult journey, I kept turning back to God. He lighted our way with the love and support He provided through visits from friends and family. As the details of my story flowed onto the paper, I noticed one of my loved ones mysteriously appeared each time I needed them most.

The visits from family and friends were helpful yet difficult at the same time. I could tell they were in shock when they saw Orion. My mom, stepfather, sisters, nephews, close friends and several members of our family called and came to show their support but no one knew what to say or do. To them, Orion seemed like a wild animal flailing all around. All I could do was tirelessly keep him from ripping out everything in sight and pray some of his energy would move to the left side of his body.

One day my friend Vita came to the hospital. As she entered the room she saw me frantically trying to control Orion. I wanted so bad to hug her but I couldn't leave my son's side. Vita is one of those friends who would come to your call at the drop of a hat, always caring and going out of her way for others. I loved her dearly. From across the room I saw deep concern in her eyes and felt her loving energy. Unfortunately, all I could do is holler from Orion's bedside, "its okay, Vita. I'll be okay." Her love and support lifted my spirits and gave me strength to get through many difficult days that followed.

Since Orion's move from the ICU, his friends were allowed to visit. Several of them came to show their support. The gesture made me realize how much my son was loved by so many. Kids he was raised with were now tall, young men and women staring in disbelief and despair. They wondered if he would ever recognize them again or if they would have to be satisfied with cherished childhood memories. I understood it was difficult for them to see Orion this way and hoped they knew how very much our family appreciated their visits.

Orion's high school film teacher, Mr. Brazell, and his class surprised us with a visit. They had made a banner and all the children signed it. Orion and I admired Mr. Brazell the kind of man who always encouraged him to pursue his passions, set goals and follow through. The two of them were very close. I could feel the sadness and see it in his eyes as he stood over Orion and talked to him that day. I was so happy to see him but couldn't seem to find the right words to say. I was just glad he had come.

Two of Orion's friends flew all the way from California to personally tell him they were there for him and praying for his recovery. Jon and Justin met Orion in college. The three of them had graduated at the same time and planned to room together as they began their careers in the film industry. My mind couldn't help but wonder if my son's dreams would ever come to pass. For now I would simply be grateful for the significant gesture of love and concern displayed by these two wonderful young men.

Another of Orion's friends, Rob, came to the hospital one day with his parents. They had been roommates at the film school and were very close friends. My mind flashed back to the two of them standing tall and proud on graduation day. But now, my heart ached for Rob as he stood over his friend's hospital bed; devastated. Rob's parents knew of Orion's love of cars and had brought him a book. It was so kind of them. I wondered if he would ever be able to read it. I tried to stay strong during their visit while we reminisced about our boys. As they were leaving I thanked them for coming and gave Rob a big hug. I could barely hold back my own tears.

It's impossible to find the right words to express our gratitude to Orion's close friends, Kelly, JT, Dante and Joey. They came to the hospital almost every day. Even though their friend looked back at them with only a blank stare, they came and reminisced about good times they had shared in the past and those yet to come. I dreamed of those future moments and prayed my dream would come true. Their support meant everything to me, and it is my hope they realize how much their presence soothed my aching soul.

My mom and sisters were always close by and did everything they could to support and comfort me. My sister Ronnie practiced massage therapy and would do reflexology on Orion to encourage healing of his body. And my mom was so supportive and there for us every day. Although she didn't know what to do as Bill and I worked with Orion's flailing body, her presence alone was comforting. My sister Debbie called daily for an updated report. She and I were very close and I knew she wanted to be here with me, but personal circumstances made it impossible. Just knowing she was only a phone call away was enough.

Bill's dad, Pop, was very close to Orion. At the time of the accident he was eighty-five years old and quite a frail man. We had tried to keep the news from him but it had been almost two months so we had to tell him of Orion's condition. Bill brought him into Orion's room. Pop's eyes filled with tears and sadness overcame him. It was such a difficult site for both of us to witness.

And then there was Grace, an amazing woman. She and I had been in spiritual teachings for many years prior to the accident. I remember she had stopped by for a visit one day and said, "While in meditation, I saw Orion riding a bike." As she spoke I looked deep into her eyes and I felt her presence inside my very being. Our souls connected for a moment and although this sounded so far out, inside somehow I knew her vision would someday come true. But how could it happen? When would it happen? Doubt tried to overtake me, but God was by my side. In my heart I knew her vision would become reality. I was afraid to mention it to anyone for fear they might think I'd lost my mind! I would push aside such useless chatter from my mind and listen to my heart. Grace's words had filled me with hope.

Days later a therapist tried to stand Orion. He looked like a noodle as his body stood limp and leaning to the left. As he attempted to put my son in a chair Orion just slid down to the floor. Seeing him this weak and frail was such a frightening and disheartening event for a mother to watch. My mind went crazy with thoughts of the unknown outcome or if my son would be labeled an invalid. In these moments of despair and confusion, it was God who eased my aching soul and redirected my thoughts to a more hopeful outcome.

These were desperate times and therefore I was open to all possibilities when it came to my son's recovery. About six weeks prior to Orion's accident, I became involved in an herbal food company. It was 'no accident' that this opportunity came into my life at that time. Grace, my sponsor and spiritual teacher, recommended I start feeding Orion these foods down his stomach tube. As I looked into her eyes I remember they gleamed with hope and encouragement. I trusted her judgment and knowledge. There was no doubt in my mind that I would make all attempts to act on her recommendation. The difficult part would be getting a doctor's order to begin feeding Orion the herbal foods, but I was determined to get it.

Shortly thereafter, I approached the first doctor with Grace's idea. He said the food was not going to help and he would not write the order. I didn't stop there. I spoke to a second doctor who said Orion's injury was too severe and the herbal food would not benefit him. He also told me I needed to face reality and start looking at nursing home placement for my son. Needless to say, that answer didn't sit well with me. Once again I moved on.

They say the third time's a charm and in my case it was. The third doctor agreed with the others that feeding my son herbal foods would not help, however he went on to say that if it would make me feel better, he would write the order.

This was all I needed to hear. The doctor wrote the order and I began feeding Orion the herbal foods down his feeding tube. I had called Grace with the good news and she gave me a list of recommended products Orion would need at this stage of his recovery. I believe our body has the capability to heal itself if given the proper nourishment. In my opinion the herbal foods would nourish my son's body, and that gave me hope for a full recovery.

I was like a mad scientist mixing, blending and pumping foods into my son in liquid form so it didn't clog the tubes. My nursing background was helpful at this point because I knew the tricks of the trade when it came to tube feeding. I was so grateful for Grace's encouraging words and confidence that the herbal foods would help nourish my son.

Swallowing was another issue. First of all, it took a couple of weeks just to get Orion to open his mouth! We were nowhere near reaching the swallowing goal because Orion still had the trache tube and his gag reflex was weak to say the least. The trache tube had to be capped off before the nurses and therapist could perform the swallow test. They would put blue dye in baby food consistency in Orion's mouth in an attempt to see if he could swallow. The test would make him gag and the contents would have to be suctioned out of his mouth. It was awful for me to watch him choke and gag but I knew it had to occur for him to regain his ability to swallow.

One evening Orion had about enough and pulled his trache tube out. The staff was shocked that someone who appeared so weak all of the sudden had the strength of Hercules. His left side still didn't budge, but his right side was obviously very strong! I could see the process of learning to swallow again was going to take a lot of time and patience.

Then there was range of motion exercises. As a nurse I understood the importance of these exercises. I had worked with stroke patients for years and was determined to do everything in my power to keep my son from developing a contracture, which is the shortening or distortion of muscular or connective tissue, or foot drop. A foot drop is weakness of muscles that are involved in flexing the ankle and toes. If Orion developed either of these two conditions, it would impede his ability to walk. My experience had taught me these were always potential problems with bed ridden patients. I worked with my son constantly while my husband and I held onto the belief he would have a full recovery. That belief is what kept us going.

Days seemed endless as Orion lay in bed. It had been seven weeks since the accident but it felt like an eternity. I stayed at his bedside stimulating his senses, moving his limbs, feeding him the herbal foods down his feeding tube, bathing him and completely caring for him. The daily regiment was similar to when he was a baby only now my son was over six feet tall, weighed 175 lbs and was twenty-one years old. How could this be happening to him? And how could this happen to our family? I pushed these thoughts aside, came to my senses and realized how fortunate we were to have him with us in any condition at all! I thanked God that Orion was alive and continued to pray for his recovery.

Did doubt continue to creep in? Yes, it did every day. Occasionally, my mind told me, "Hey, who are you fooling? You're a nurse. You know the extent of his injury." But then my heart spoke of something quite different. My heart knew intuitively that I had to keep trying. No matter how it looked on the outside or what the doctors said, I felt his prognosis would be that somehow he would get through this. I held tightly onto hope and my faith in God. I made myself get out of my 'head' and go to my 'heart' because that's where the true answer lies.

This was definitely the hardest thing I had ever been through! But I had help. I could not have done it without the love, presence and support of God, my friends and family. It was more comforting than they could have imagined. To this day, it sends chills down my spine.

INPATIENT REHABILITATION THERAPY

After a lengthy stay in the hospital Orion was discharged to a rehabilitation hospital for inpatient therapy. It was time for the next phase of his journey to recovery. I was extremely nervous because I didn't know what to expect. As preparations were being made my anxiety was overwhelming. I was excited to get my son out of the hospital, but I didn't know how to handle all of these emotions; fear, anxiety, relief. I lived in a state of uncertainty, but vowed to continue pushing forward, one day at a time, God by my side.

Orion would be transported to the new facility. As we waited for the driver I tried to explain to my son that we were going to a new hospital for therapy. He still had a trache tube as his airway and a feeding tube. He was very weak, could barely hold up his head and his left side was still flaccid. Orion's limited communication skills consisted of words spelled out using the alphabet board and his thumb up/down signals as he could not yet speak. Although his condition probably seemed awful to strangers it was glorious to me! He had come such a long way from his life threatening, comatose state following the accident. I was grateful to see my son alive and alert as we exited the hospital.

When the driver arrived he was very cheerful and asked Orion what kind of music he liked. The driver mentioned country music and a few others, but Orion kept giving him thumbs down. Finally, Orion spelled out 'Led Zeppelin' on his alphabet board. This was the only music he and his Dad had in common. The driver smiled and said, "Zeppelin it is!" He and an assistant moved Orion to the stretcher and off they went. Bill and I followed, driving more than an hour and a half before reaching our destination.

When we arrived at the rehabilitation facility it was unfamiliar and frightening. There were people strapped to wheelchairs, some yelling, others drooling. Although I didn't really know what to expect I wasn't prepared to see this. Nor was I convinced I wanted to move my son to this kind of environment. I had to stay strong and believe this was all part of God's divine plan. He had brought us to this place and I had to trust His guidance.

Shortly after Orion was settled in his room we were greeted by a friendly staff and my anxiety soon settled. A nurse sat down with us and attempted to go over Orion's goals during his stay. As she went through the list, all Orion could do was spell out the word D-R-I-V-E over and over again on his letter board. The nurse looked astonished to see this weak young man, still unable to hold up his head or walk, wanting his only goal to be to drive again. Orion always loved to drive. He loved cars as much as his brother loved surfboards. The nurse said, "Well, young man, let's try to get you walking first." Orion once again impatiently spelled out D-R-I-V-E. That appeared to be his only desire. In his mind we could just skip all the walking, talking, bathing and feeding himself. Orion wanted to get straight to the 'good stuff,' driving.

In my heart I felt some relief because I knew my son was still in this body as his passion for driving was still apparent. At the same time I did not know if we could make his dream come true. As Orion impatiently kept spelling out D-R- I-V-E on the letter board, I said, "Son, you will drive again someday, but for now let's see if we can get you walking first." He once again spelled D-R-I-V-E. The nurse laughed and said "Boy, he sure is determined. And that's a good thing!" I agreed. After all, he needed that motivation to continue moving forward. Orion's determination was encouraging and lifted my spirits. My skepticism had transitioned to hope.

As dusk fell and we settled in for the night we heard a lady across the hall relentlessly yelling, "Help me!" I asked the nurse if she was okay and was told she usually screams all night. Orion, with his crooked smile, looked at me as if to say, 'Oh boy. Here we go. It's going to be a long night!' His sense of humor had begun to surface and raised my spirits to new heights.

We needed a diversion from the screaming. I remembered when Orion had been in the coma we were told to play classical music in his room. We understood it to be from the masters of music which was close to God. That evening he drifted off to sleep with the beautiful sound of *Beethoven* playing in the background.

The night was long with nurses coming in and out the room. They checked his vital signs, pupils and administered medicine in his feeding tube. Then they would ask him questions to see if his responses were appropriate. Orion would respond with thumbs up/down communication. He would doze off to sleep only to have the nurse's aide come in to see if he needed to be turned or propped to the other side. Once again, he settled down to sleep while the screams from across the hall continued, "Help me! Help me!" The experience saddened my heart. I slept very little due to the uncertainty of this new stage of our journey. It left me very unsettled inside yet I had to appear strong for Orion's sake. I couldn't let him know how afraid and alone I felt.

The next morning with little sleep under our belts, we were greeted by the Occupational Therapist. She was a spunky young woman with a lot of energy. Her first order of business was to see how much Orion could accomplish without help. I was asked only to observe. As a mother, this was not an easy thing to do! However I stepped back and watched as the therapist handed Orion his pants and asked him to put them on. There was such determination on his face as he tugged and pulled, struggling with his non-dominant hand to pull them up. Several minutes later he had them part way up and backward, but it was a good start. The shirt was even more of a challenge. I had forgotten how difficult a supposedly simple task could be. It was like a flashback in time to my child learning to dress himself. Another twenty minutes or so later he had it on. The shirt was inside out and his arm was in the hole where the head goes and vice versa. Sweat was pouring from Orion's brow and I could see the frustration in his eyes. To stand by and helplessly watch him struggle through this exercise was very difficult, but I knew it had to be done for the therapist to evaluate his condition and for my son to learn.

Later in the day the doctor arrived. He determined that Orion's oxygen level had stabilized during the course of the last several days, so he would remove his trache tube. This was a tremendous step forward! I was thrilled and nervous at the same time. Without the trache the staff would have to constantly monitor Orion's oxygen levels and administer oxygen if they fell below an acceptable reading. Occasionally I would witness the O2 Sat monitor (the machine that monitors the oxygen levels) drop below an acceptable number and would encourage Orion to take a deep breath. My anxiety eased during the course of the next few days as he was able to completely wean off the oxygen altogether. He had overcome yet another hurdle.

Orion's progress was slow. Nonetheless, Bill and I, along with the therapists, worked relentlessly with him and I continued to religiously feed him the herbal foods, never missing a meal. There were little signs of further improvement, but we were determined to get our son back. His recovery had become our purpose for living.

I would do *anything* in my power to make my son better. I mixed the herbal foods and put them in his feeding tube faithfully, bathed him in holy water that a friend brought by and called in holistic healers. I even had a Buddhist monk come in to recite sacred healing chants. There were prayers being said all over the world to help our son. At one point, my mom made the comment, "You even have the atheist praying." I tried everything because deep inside I knew that positive, healing energy was so important for our miracle to happen. It was the most difficult time of my life, but I wouldn't give up.

This was just the beginning of Orion's rehabilitation. He would undergo multiple therapy sessions each and every day for weeks during his stay in the rehab facility. Occupational Therapy (OT) was used to teach him to perform activities of daily living, including dressing and feeding himself, combing his hair, brushing his teeth and tying his shoes. Twenty-one years of daily skills had to be taught, practiced and achieved throughout these sessions and the following months. And he would have to master most of these skills with his one non-dominant hand. There would be many bumps and bends along the way long road to recovery.

Physical Therapy (PT) was designed to help Orion with his balance, strength and coordination. These sessions included activities such as mat exercises to strengthen his legs. Each day two therapists assisted him, one on each side to help him balance and move one foot in front of the other. The ultimate goal was to teach my son to walk again but at this stage he was even too weak to hold his body up without assistance from the therapists.

Days turned into weeks while I watched in anticipation as my son worked so hard to make progress. Sweat poured from his weak body throughout each session. While one therapist braced him on the bars he took a step with his right leg. Then another therapist moved his left leg forward. When he reached the end of the walk he looked over to me as if to say, 'Are you taking notes?' He was so determined and I was so proud of him. I watched every session with hopes that someday my son would be able to walk again. And yes, I took notes. Orion made sure of it!

One morning before our daily routine started, Orion was sleeping, so I went to start some laundry at the station down the hall. I returned to his room about the same time that the OT therapist arrived. The room was in shambles! There was Orion lying in the bed, yet there were things thrown all about. He muttered, "I just walked to the bathroom." The therapist and I looked at each other, confused. Somehow, Orion had managed to get out of bed and go to the bathroom, knocking down everything in his path. The therapist said, "Well, let's get you up and walking then." She sent an assistant to locate a 'quad cane' and bring it back to the room. Orion's legs wobbled as the therapist attempted to stand him. When he saw the cane he said, "Get that old man cane away from me!" The therapist smiled as if to say, "It's going to be a challenging day."

Orion also attended Individual and group Speech Therapy (ST) sessions. It is common for TBI patients to have voice issues that the speech therapist addresses, along with teaching them to swallow, as well as performing ongoing mouth exercises to regain his smile. After Orion's trache was removed, part of these sessions also focused on speaking exercises to create voice inflection because he spoke in a completely monotone voice.

The most important goal in ST was to teach Orion to swallow since he was still receiving his nutrition through his feeding tube. To do this he practiced throat exercises to strengthen his gag reflex. The therapists fed him very small amounts of various food consistencies to prepare him for his weekly swallow test. They worked diligently with him while he choked and gagged. This was one of the most difficult things to watch. I was anxious for the day his feeding tube could be removed and he could eat and drink again.

Cognitive Therapy (CT) worked with Orion's memory which was extremely affected by the accident. He was unable to remember things from one day to the next including the date, president, and other commonly known information. Orion suffered from impulsivity as well, which meant he was inclined to act on impulse rather than thought. This condition is very common among TBI patients and made it even more challenging for my son to improve his cognitive skills.

Orion's CT therapist had boards covered with lights. When a light flashed on, Orion would hit the light as quickly as he could, working to improve his response time. In the beginning his reaction was very slow. A light on the board would flash but he was unable to hit it before the next one came on. I saw the frustration on his face. The exercise took a lot of patience and improvement in this area didn't happen overnight. In fact, it was weeks before I saw any progress. Eventually he was able to successfully perform the exercise.

The CT therapists also told Orion stories and later asked him questions to test his memory skills. In time, his replies improved and became more accurate. In the beginning the therapist would read a short story and then immediately ask him simple questions. So many thoughts raced through my mind as I sat quietly awaiting his response. This exercise appeared to be a basic memory game yet it was several weeks before I observed improvements in this area. I admired my son's persistence and patience.

Recreational Therapy (RT) began after Orion had progressed about a month into the other therapies. RT consists of just what it sounds like, Recreation. I rolled his wheelchair into the recreation room where various activities took place. One day a very outgoing young girl said "Come on, Orion. You're not going to let a girl beat you, are you?" The game involved throwing sandbags in a hole, and Orion used his right arm to take on the challenge. When he finally put one in the hole, I don't know who was happier, the girl or me. We both yelled "Yeah!" No girl was going to beat him! I saw his crooked little smile and could tell this small victory would make him try even harder. My son was getting better with every session as the weeks passed. His coordination improved tremendously during this time, giving all of us hope that he would recover.

Orion's feeding tube had been removed from his stomach after the first couple weeks at the rehab facility. Yet another miracle had happened. I gave thanks to God and prayed for strength. Now I was feeding my son baby food and wondering how in the world I was going to handle this. And am I strong enough to hold on? Then those precious words would return to my mind, "With God, all things are possible." With Him by my side I could do anything.

After a full day of therapy sessions I rolled Orion's wheelchair outside by the lake and started the exercises all over again. He insisted that I take notes in all the sessions so I pulled them out and said, "Well what are you waiting for? No slacking on my watch." That seemed to be just what he wanted to hear. We smiled at each other and at that moment I felt as if it was somehow going to be okay. I didn't know how or even question my feelings. It just felt right. I hoped I could maintain this peaceful mood as I sat under the oak tree by my son's side. We spent hours practicing facial exercises to try and regain his beautiful smile. We stuck out our tongues at one another and practiced the mouth exercises over and over again. People walked by and stared at us, but in my mind nothing else mattered but getting my son's smile and voice back.

Big, bright-red goldfish type fish swam in the lake beside us. I would point out the fish to my son, but in his blank stare I knew he couldn't see. Orion was born with a cataract in his left eye. He underwent surgery at about sixteen months old to correct the problem. The procedure was called *Epikeratophakia*. My husband and I were told this procedure would not help his condition at an older age, so we agreed to the surgery. A donor lens was sewed onto the outside of the eye and afterwards a patch was placed on his right eye to force him to see out of his left eye. This was not always an easy task with a rambunctious toddler! As fate would have it, we lived on a sailboat so the patch over his eye fit right in with our lifestyle. I saw the inquisitive looks on stranger's faces as they walked by the boat and heard remarks such as 'Oh isn't that cute honey. They dress their son like a pirate.' Their comments didn't bother me. He was my little pirate and he meant the world to both his father and I.

The doctor used the surgery and a patch on his right eye in an effort to cause light to stimulate Orion's use of his left eye. As a result of this birth defect, Orion had poor vision in his left eye and was legally blind in that eye since birth. This was the reason he could not see the goldfish in the lake. To make matters worse, the vision in his right eye had been affected by the accident. I knew vision was often affected in brain injured patients but later I discovered that it was more common than not.

Each day was a challenge for me because Orion couldn't remember from day to day what had happened. Nor could he remember anyone's name, the date, or the accident itself. It was as if every day was a new beginning for my son. Before we left his room, I would drill him for the day. My hope was that he would still remember the day's events by the time we made it to the end of the hallway. We went over the name of the president, the season, days of the week, the month, day and year, etc. We reviewed the same facts day after day only for him to forget everything by the time we reached the therapy session. My heart was breaking but I couldn't show Orion that part of me. Even though my family and friends were there for me, I felt so afraid and alone at times. I wanted our old life back, but as I was now well aware, it was forever changed.

I remember one OT session when the therapist rolled Orion into the gift shop and told him to buy some peanut M&M's. I was shocked to realize that he couldn't see the bright yellow bags right in front of his face. When it came time to pay for the candy he couldn't recognize the difference between a quarter and a dime. This was difficult to watch, but I was determined that my son, a college graduate, always on the honor role and a brilliant young man, could buy a bag of peanut M&M's. I thought, what in the world are we going to do? I remembered Orion really liked one of his therapists. She was a sweet, young girl named Georgia. Even though he didn't remember her from day to day, his eyes would light up whenever she worked with him. And guess what? She loved peanut M&M's.

Although I wasn't sure if he was allowed to venture from the rehab facility property, I rolled Orion in his wheelchair to a nearby drug store. As we made our way to the candy aisle, I told him to buy Georgia, the young female therapist, some M&M's. I agreed to pay for the candy if he picked them out. I watched him, barely able to hold up his head or his body, scan the aisle for the big, bright yellow bag.

After what seemed like over an hour, Orion finally found them. I lit up like a lighthouse and said, "You did it! I knew you could do it!" While I sometimes felt as if my whole world was being ripped apart, I began to find life's pleasures in the little things. My twenty-one year old son could pick out a yellow bag of peanut M&M's. I couldn't wait for the next day when he could give them to his therapist.

The following morning I reminded Orion of the therapist's name and the M&Ms before we went into the session. Amazingly, he seemed to remember! Orion anxiously smiled when she walked into the room and immediately handed her the bag of candy. She was so pleased! The look of accomplishment on my son's face was something I will never forget. This was yet another small step in his journey.

Hours seemed like days and the tears came and went as I sat through every therapy session. During the group speech sessions Orion was placed in front of a mirror to perform certain mouth exercises, such as stick his tongue out and practice saying words. We would roll in daily, his mouth drooping while I tried to wipe away the drool. The group consisted of about five to six older patients, mostly stroke victims. I can't tell you how hard it was to push my son's wheelchair up next to them. It just seemed so unfair! He's only twenty-one years old. I thought to myself, this thing doesn't happen until a person's in his or her seventies or eighties, right? I felt as if my young son did not belong there, but I knew in my heart this was one of many critical stops on his road to recovery.

The difference in past and present reasoning is very evident in TBI patients. The physiologist told us this self-awareness issue in Orion was a big factor. He said that when the frontal lobe is damaged, a person's awareness of his or her past and present thinking is greatly different, yet the patient does not realize it. Orion didn't recognize his mental and sometimes even physical changes easily spotted by someone else. This was very apparent when Orion believed he could perform his filming job today, just as he had prior to the accident.

Orion attended a very prominent film school and had been assisting with filming independent and even a few large scale film projects prior to his injury. Shortly before the accident he had turned down a very good job to work on some personal projects he was pursuing. After the accident, Orion did not understand that he was no longer capable of performing at that level.

The OT therapist believed getting Orion to simulate filming one of the sessions would spark some interest in him, and it did! Someone graciously donated a hand held movie camera for Orion to use in therapy. When the therapist suggested Orion film the session, my husband saw life come back into his eyes and an expression of happiness appear on his face. Most of the time Orion was unemotional in these sessions, but this had genuinely sparked him back into life. Bill sensed his son felt alive, hopeful and filled with the usefulness that is sometimes taken away when a person is told that what he or she loves to do is no longer possible.

The joy of seeing Orion's enthusiasm quickly disappeared when it was apparent that physically and mentally he was not going to be able to film the session. In our judgments of others we sometimes forget that with a positive attitude and faith, all things are possible. Hope and faith are sometimes hard to hold on to when we judge with our human emotions. What Bill saw crushed him and made him so sad. Although tears filled my husband's eyes as he told me the story, he couldn't show Orion his pain and didn't want to feel it, but it was there. Our son couldn't figure out how to put the film in the camera, turn it on, hold it steady or even point it in the right direction. As we had been warned, these things didn't bother Orion. What others saw as a failed attempt was a complete success to him.

My husband began believing some of the things the doctors had been telling us; he'll never work, take care of himself, or live on his own, even though he had already accomplished so many things he wasn't supposed to be able to do. Bill tried not to look in a negative way, but instead went back to his thinking that it's all okay. He had to remind himself to stop judging and just keep looking for miracles, for he knew they would appear. Maybe not the way he wanted them to, but according to God's plan. He smiled and said, "Good job!" to his son. My heart burst with love for my husband. I smiled and gave his hand a squeeze, knowing it's what he needed in that moment.

I was blessed with two beautiful sons and I missed Noah, my younger son, dearly every moment of every day. There wasn't a day that went by that I didn't think about him, but I knew I had to spend my time working with Orion. I wanted my family back the way it was before. It didn't seem fair that I was placed in this difficult circumstance. I struggled with why God would let this happen. Even worse, I questioned if it was my fault in some way? Our minds sometimes play tricks on us when we lack sleep and feel the frustration from weeks of separation from our loved ones. In such moments I had to hold on to my faith and remember, 'With God, all things are possible.' I would have my family back again. I prayed for patience and the strength to achieve that goal.

Day after day of intense therapy continued and it wasn't getting any easier. I cried several times a day, in private, while trying to stay strong in front of Orion. Inside I felt as if someone had ripped my heart out. My son, once strong and healthy, was now so fragile. In family counseling I realized I was not alone. There were five other mothers whose children had Traumatic Brain Injuries and they were just as devastated as I was.

Then one day Orion tried to talk to me. I could barely understand his unfamiliar voice which was very frustrating for both of us. The left side of his mouth drooped and he drooled as he attempted to speak, but I thought, "Wow! He can talk!" In a soft, slurred voice, Orion said, "My voice sucks." I replied, "Son, two days ago you couldn't speak. Your voice sounds beautiful to me!" The left side of a person's brain houses the language centers, and shortly after the accident we were told he would never be able to talk. Orion proved them wrong. He was talking! It was music to my ears.

Shortly after his first words, there was another significant day. We were in the dining room and I was feeding Orion. I asked him if he would like some more mashed potatoes. He replied, "How can I have more, when I haven't had *any* yet?" He was right and went on to say, "Don't worry mom, it's only a technicality." At that moment I knew that my intelligent son was still there! He was reasoning with me. I knew my son was on his way back to us. It was a mother's intuition, something no words could ever fully describe. I believe intuition to be divine guidance; the God within talking to us on a deeper level. Our intuition is God's way of guiding us to the right path. It's that inner knowledge or gut feeling that will always guide us to the right path if we learn to trust it.

Using words like 'technicality' was an amazing accomplishment. I had noticed other patients having difficulty finding much smaller words. Prior to the accident, Orion's vocabulary had always been excellent. I realized if he was using big words like this then he was going to be fine! Moments like these kept me going.

Little did I know there would be yet another roadblock when I arrived the next morning. I sat across from the social worker who told me she did not know how much more therapy my son would be able to attend because our insurance was reaching the maximum. My voice trembled as I began to plead my case. I said, "You don't understand, my son's still in there. He said the word 'technicality' last night." My eyes filled with tears as I went on to tell her that I had to do everything possible to continue his recovery program. I wondered if anyone else could see Orion's progress or was I just dreaming a pipe dream? Or did I just sound like a desperate mother striving to get one last chance to save her son? I didn't know.

The next day we met again. This time the meeting included the entire family, the social worker, the therapists, and the doctor. The therapists each took their turn presenting my son's progress. Then the social worker and family members spoke about their concerns. Finally it was my turn. I described Orion's progress from my perspective and that I knew he would continue to make progress if given the chance. I went on to plead my case by complimenting the facility and staff. It was my understanding the rehabilitation facility was well known for their expertise and our experience with my son's team of therapists confirmed that fact. They were skilled and devoted employees. Orion had made tremendous progress to date and he and the team were working exceptionally well together in my opinion. The social worker mentioned that their charity fund had some money still available for the year. Our family had never accepted charity before but my pride was the last thing I was worried about at a time like this. We humbly welcomed their donation. I was extremely nervous as I sat in the room anxiously awaiting the teams reply. At last they came forward with their decision. The therapy would continue for two more weeks and Orion's case would be reevaluated at that time. We were humbled and very grateful.

We continued our daily therapy routine through the remainder of Orion's stay at the rehab facility. It consisted of sessions throughout the day, each one lasting thirty to forty-five minutes. Our day started early at 7:00 a.m. when I would wake him up and change his wet clothing if necessary. Next I would get the breakfast setup and work with my son to practice feeding himself. After breakfast I would watch as he attempted to get dressed and then help him along so he was ready in time for the first session. The therapist would arrive and instruct him on how to transfer from the bed to the wheelchair. Orion would make valiant attempts, but his weak body would not cooperate. After all, it had been months since he last used his body to move around. He was definitely improving. The process was just going to take some time. The therapist and I would then roll him into the bathroom, hand him a toothbrush and water as he attempted to find his mouth and brush his teeth. At last we were off to tackle a full day's schedule.

I would take notes in all the sessions and sit patiently waiting to ask questions. After the day's therapy sessions ended, Orion and I would go through the exercises again, over and over, by the lake, in the room, in the lounge or under the oak tree. We were so determined to succeed. Orion worked feverishly in all the therapy sessions as I stood back and admired his persistence in action. We were fortunate that Orion's injury did not seem to affect his ability to initiate activities as is the case with some TBI patients. Instead, he listened intently to all instructions and immediately began to perfect each movement.

At this point Orion was really working on his swallowing. One day in his speech session, the therapist said she would put a little cola on the straw to see if he could tolerate it. He was always a 'label guy', and sure enough, out she came with a generic brand. Orion's face grimaced with the taste as he began choking and gagging. I mentioned to the therapist that as silly as it sounded I thought Orion would do better with a name brand. She told me there was no difference, but I offered to purchase one and give it a try. The next day we once again attempted with the 'real McCoy.' He still gagged, but I could tell he tolerated it much better.

That night Noah talked to him as I held the phone to Orion's ear. They made a pact. Noah would not have a cola until his brother was able to swallow. I was so proud of Noah! He was doing anything he could to help his brother get well. The bond between them was as strong as when they were young boys.

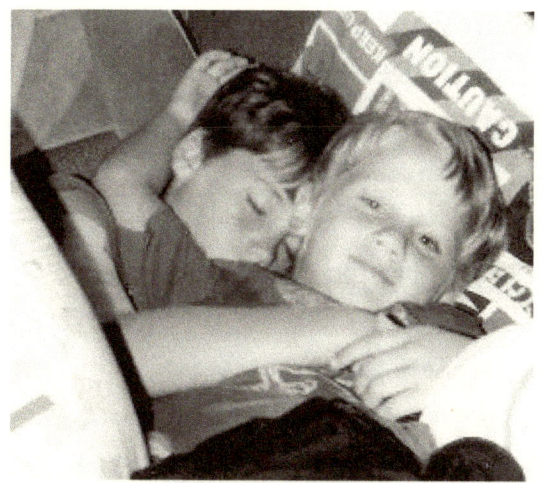

Orion and Noah

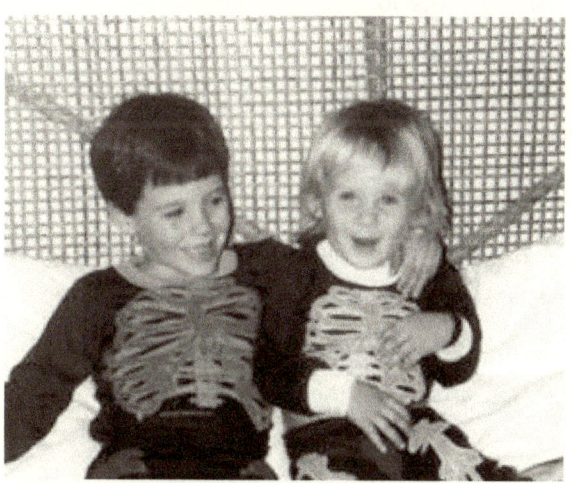

My boys in their glow-in-the-dark skeleton PJ's

Orion's various therapies continued. One day as we proceeded through our daily regimen of sessions, Orion sat on a mat with the physical therapist. He used his right hand to help steady himself because he was not able to maintain a posture or move his left side without help from his other side. He did whatever it took to make his left side move, even if he had to cheat and use the right side. The therapist said, "Orion, look at your left arm. Now concentrate and see if you can move it." Orion looked intently at his left arm. I saw the focus and determination on his face but the arm just lay there, motionless. Just as I began to wonder if this challenge was too difficult, he took his right hand and moved the left arm just where the therapist had said to put it and looked back at him as if to say, 'There you go.' Orion would not be defeated. As a tribute to his constant innovation and determination the therapist gave him the title, *master of compensation*. The look on my son's face mirrored that of an Olympic champion. He was so proud of his achievement and the new title that came with it.

Orion's inner drive and determination was like no other. Throughout the daily therapy sessions, he would give me the 'Are you taking notes' look because he knew after the sessions concluded, we would repeat the day's exercises. In fact, there were days he had more energy that I did; and he was the patient!

As he progressed, the therapists attempted to get him to stand and begin to walk. They would brace him on both sides, move the left leg and prompt him to take a step. It was like teaching a 6' 1" toddler to walk. As a mother, watching my son struggle was very difficult, but I could see him getting stronger. He was slowly on his way to walking again! I was so grateful and amazed as I witnessed God's miracle in action.

Orion and I continued to work hard before, during, and after sessions. I would mix the packets of herbal foods and make sure he was fed three times a day. I had a toddler again, and even though he was over six feet tall and weighed 175 lbs., he was my son and I would do anything to get him back. He was eager to learn, like a child learning to walk. You could see it in his eyes. So I requested pool therapy for Orion. The water would be good for his body and perhaps more like play than the grueling therapy regiment.

His first day of pool therapy was a terrifying for me. Every mother understands the fear of when young children head for the water's edge and mine was no different. Orion's weak, limp body didn't want to cooperate all the time, so the process of getting him in the pool was itself quite difficult. A special water boot was designed for the occasion. It kept his left foot steady and straight. As we placed him in the shallow pool of water, his body relaxed and seemed to flow much easier than it did out of the water.

Of course, mom got to go in the water too. It was wonderful! Orion's eyes sparkled like I hadn't seen in a very long time as he floated and the therapist guided his hand across the water. He seemed to become a part of the water as his arms and legs floated. His body was so loose and flexible, flowing freely in the water as the therapist guided him. This new therapy choice was so good for Orion and for me as well. Apart from the mundane, daily therapies, this was fun! We seemed to let it all go that day. The pool therapy would become an addition to our daily routine. Today, we let our cares float away.

The sessions continued until one day the therapist said, "Okay, mom. He's all yours." I was anxious and scared at the same time. What if I couldn't handle him? What if he slipped and maybe drowned? How can I do this? As I took his body in mine and guided him with a gentle motion through the water, those fears floated away. God was with us. I felt it. There was nothing to be afraid of. We floated from one side to the other as I gently directed his weak side to promote the range of motion. It was so much easier in the water. His left side glided effortlessly through the water with my guidance.

As we floated in the pool, I drifted back in time to when he was two years old and had his first swimming lesson. Orion was much bigger now, of course, but this was still my child regardless of age or size. The excitement in his bright eyes was the same today. We finished our session and couldn't wait until the next one. The therapist lifted Orion out of the pool with a special chair lift and I snuggled him in a large, warm towel. He was still glowing, and so was I. For the first time since that fateful day on April 2nd, I smiled. I wouldn't judge it, but rather bask in the joy and peace of the moment.

Back at the room, I dried Orion's hair, changed his clothes and fell back to the routine. It was time for a parent's session, so I gently tucked him in, made sure all his bedrails were positioned and explained I would be back in fifteen minutes. I knew he would sleep after such an invigorating therapy session.

As I approached the parent session, I noticed four women and a therapist. It seemed odd there were no fathers present. Then I remembered the reality was they had to maintain the home front while the mothers cared for the injured child. A mother has such a unique and special connection with her children. After all, we carry them for nine months and the bonding begins before they are even born. It made sense that only women were present. The looks on the mother's faces were that of fear, anxiety and uncertainty. I understood. I had the same look on mine.

The group therapist spoke of statistics associated with brain injury and how young males were most susceptible. I thought, 'Who needs statistics?' This was the last thing I needed to hear. The session was going to be depressing. As she went on to discuss the areas of the brain, we wrote feverishly and tried to grasp which part reflected our child's injury. We strived to understand as the therapist proceeded to explain the cognitive and physical changes our beloved children were experiencing. One very meaningful statistic that stuck in my mind was that it was estimated 1.5 million people sustain TBI annually. Hearing the statistic still didn't ease my pain but at least I knew I wasn't the only one going through this. I was both shocked and saddened by the information.

The following statistics from the Centers for Disease Control include the estimates of the prevalence of TBI I feel it really paints a clear picture of how big this problem really is. And to further worsen the situation, the chart that follows documents the annual TBI injuries have grown from 1.5 million to 1.7 million as of 2012.

Comparision of Annual Incidence

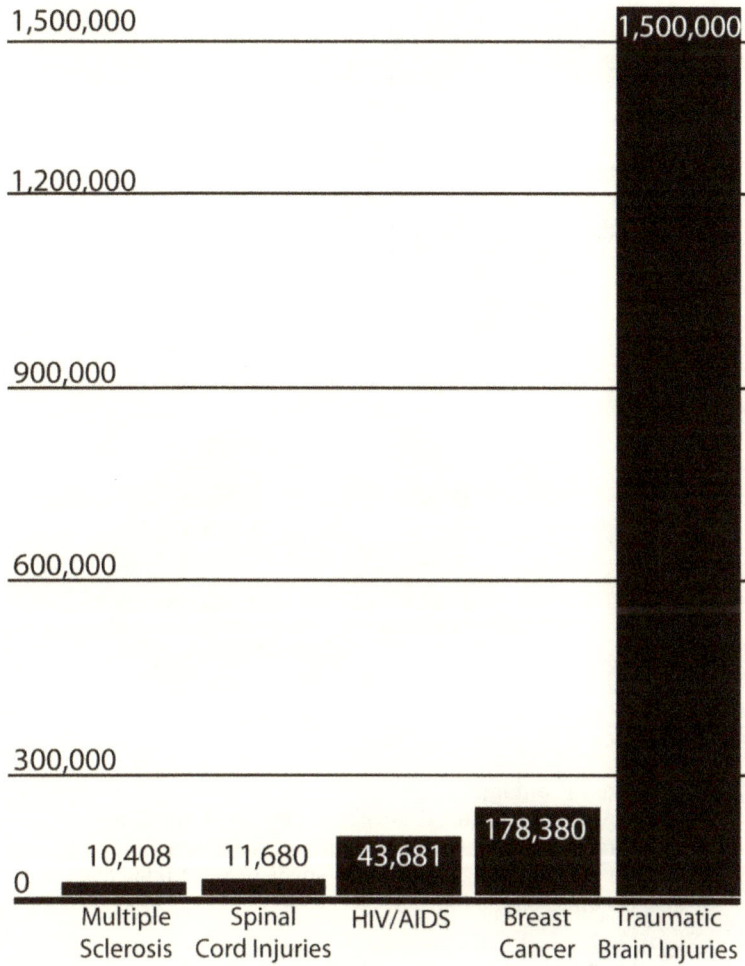

Source:
The Essential Brain Injury Guide, 4th Edition. Copyright 2007, American Academy for the Certification of Brain Injury Specialists, Brain Injury Association of America. Used by permission.

The charts on the following pages contain current statistics about the *causes and facts* of Traumatic Brain Injury.

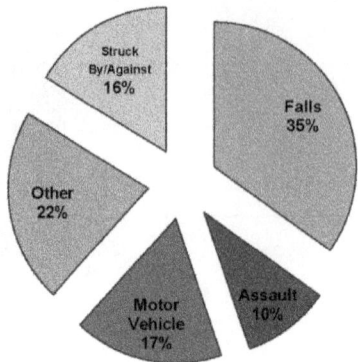

Typical Causes of TBI

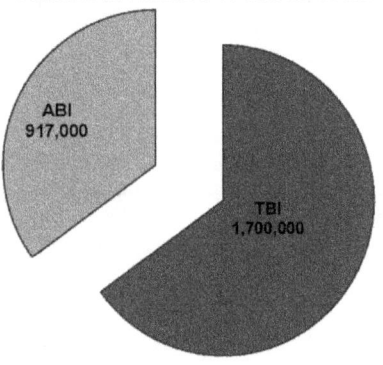

Annual Incidence of TBI and ABI

Acquired Brain Injury (ABI)
An acquired brain injury is an injury to the brain, which is not hereditary, congenital, degenerative, or induced by birth trauma. An acquired brain injury is an injury to the brain that has occurred after birth.

Type of Acquired Brain Injury	Estimated Annual Incidence
Stroke	795,000
Tumor	64,530
Aneurysm	27,000
Viral Encephalitis	20,000
Multiple Sclerosis	10,400
Anoxic/Hypoxic	No National Data Available

Facts about Brain Injury
- 5.3 million Americans live with a long-term disability as a result of TBI.
- Motor vehicle crashes and traffic-related incidences are the cause of 31.8% of TBI deaths.
- Males are more likely than females to sustain a TBI at any age.
- 75% of traumatic brain injuries are classified as "mild."
- The annual cost of TBI to society exceeds $76.5 billion.
- The estimated cost of stroke in the United States was $53.9 billion in 2010.
- In 2005, nearly 1.1 million stroke survivors reported difficulty performing basic activities of daily life.

References

Central Brain Tumor Registry of the United States (CBTRUS). CBTRUS statistical report: primary brain and central nervous system tumors diagnosed in the United States in 2004-2008. Hinsdale (IL): Central Brain Tumor Registry of the United States; 2012, Feb.

Centers for Disease Control and Prevention (CDC). Information on Arboviral Encephalitis. Atlanta (GA): Centers for Disease Control and Prevention; 2005, Nov.

Centers for Disease Control and Prevention (CDC). Prevalence and most common causes of disability among adults—United States, 2005. MMWR 2009; 58(16):421–426.

Centers for Disease Control and Prevention (CDC), National Center for Injury Prevention and Control. Report to Congress on mild traumatic brain injury in the United States: steps to prevent a serious public health problem. Atlanta (GA): Centers for Disease Control and Prevention; 2003.

Center for Disease Control and Prevention (CDC). National Center for Injury Prevention and Control. Report to Congress on traumatic brain injury in the United States. Atlanta (GA): Centers for Disease Control and Prevention; 1999, Dec.

Coronado, McGuire, Faul, Sugerman, Pearson. The epidemiology and prevention of TBI (in press) 2012.

Faul M, Xu L, Wald MM, Coronado VG. Traumatic brain injury in the United States: emergency department visits, hospitalizations, and deaths. Atlanta (GA): Centers for Disease Control and Prevention, National Center for Injury Prevention and Control; 2010.

Finkelstein E, Corso P, Miller T and associates. The incidence and economic burden of injuries in the United States. New York (NY): Oxford University Press; 2006.

National Heart Blood and Lung Institute. National Institutes of Health. What is an Aneurysm? Bethesda (Md.): National Institutes of Health; 2011.

Roger VL, Go AS, Lloyd-Jones DM, et al. Heart disease and stroke statistics—2011 update: a report from the American Heart Association. Circulation. 2011 Feb. 1; 123(4):e18-e209. Epub 2010 Dec.15.

Source: Brain Injury Association of America. (2012). In *Brain Injury Facts* find *Brain Injury Statistics*. Retrieved June 13, 2012.
www.biausa.org/Default.aspx?PageID=3599264&A=SearchResult&SearchID=4388829&ObjectID=3599264&ObjectType=1

The next part of the class was nearly more than I could bear. The therapist pointed out Orion's injury and said it was the most severe of all the patients and that multiple areas of his brain were affected. Tears flowed from my eyes, as well as the eyes of others. I attempted to scribble more notes but struggled to comprehend all of the information being presented, I was overcome with grief as were the rest of the mothers in the class. Understandably we took away very little from the class due to the emotionally stressful content. But everyone released a lot of emotion during that session.

As I left the parent session, I noticed a chart on the wall that described the differences between left- and right-sided injuries. Looking over the list of cognitive deficits, I saw that Orion's symptoms were all noted as right-sided injury. This was confusing as it was opposite of the charts. Typically, when a person's injury is on the left side of the head, the right side of the body is paralyzed and vice versa. This was not the case with Orion. The left side of his brain was injured in the accident and the left side of his body was most affected by the injury.

The following information is from the Brain Injury Association of America website and describes the functions associated with the right and left sides of the brain.

RIGHT OR LEFT BRAIN?

The functional sections or lobes of the brain are also divided into right and left sides. The right side and the left side of the brain are responsible for different functions. General patterns of dysfunction can occur if an injury is on the right or left side of the brain.

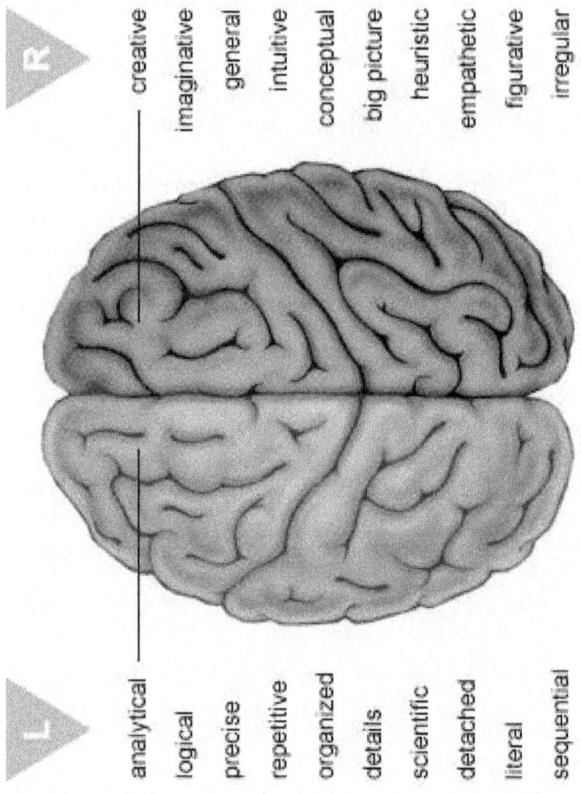

Injuries of the left side of the brain can cause:

- Difficulties in understanding language (receptive language)
- Difficulties in speaking or verbal output (expressive language)
- Catastrophic reactions (depression, anxiety)
- Verbal memory deficits
- Impaired logic
- Sequencing difficulties
- Decreased control over right-sided body movements

Injuries of the right side of the brain can cause:

- Visual-spatial impairment
- Visual memory deficits
- Left neglect (inattention to the left side of the body)
- Decreased awareness of deficits
- Altered creativity and music perception
- Loss of "the big picture" type of thinking
- Decreased control over left-sided body movements

Diffuse Brain Injury (The injuries are scattered throughout both sides of the brain) can cause:

- Reduced thinking speed
- Confusion
- Reduced attention and concentration
- Fatigue
- Impaired cognitive (thinking) skills in all areas

Source: Nucleus Medical Media. (2009). Living *with Brain Injury*. Retrieved June 13, 2012. www.biausa.org/living-with-brain-injury.htm

The doctors told us that Orion most likely suffered a *contrecoup* injury meaning the tissue damage is on the side opposite the trauma site. They went on to explain that a *contrecoup* injury occurs when the head stops abruptly at impact and the brain collides with the inside of the skull. The doctors also indicated Orion had several small bleeds throughout his brain including the frontal, parietal and temporal lobes, but the major bleed was the left hemisphere. The only important thing to his father and I was that our son was learning to talk, write, dress himself and function using his right hand. This was a difficult endeavor as he was left-handed prior to the accident.

The following information is from the Brain Injury Association of America website and outlines the parts of the brain and the functions they perform.

FUNCTIONS OF THE BRAIN

The brain is divided into main functional sections, called lobes. These sections or brain lobes are called the Frontal Lobe, Temporal Lobe, Parietal Lobe, Occipital Lobe, the Cerebellum, and the Brain Stem. Each has a specific function as described below.

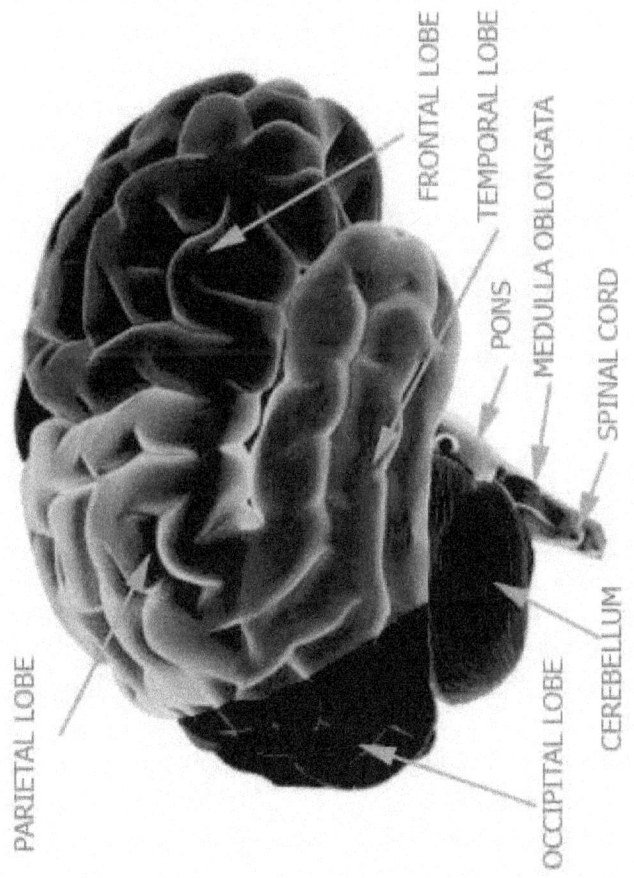

Parietal Lobe Functions

- Sense of touch
- Spatial perception
- Differentiation (identification) of size, shapes, and colors
- Visual perception

Occipital Lobe Functions

- Vision

Cerebellum Lobe Functions

- Balance
- Skilled motor activity
- Coordination
- Visual perception

Brain Stem Functions

- Breathing
- Arousal and consciousness
- Attention and concentration
- Heart rate
- Sleep and wake cycles

Frontal Lobe Functions

- Attention and concentration
- Self-monitoring
- Organization
- Speaking (expressive language)
- Motor planning and initiation
- Awareness of abilities and limitations
- Personality
- Mental flexibility
- Inhibition of behavior
- Emotions
- Problem solving
- Planning and anticipation
- Judgment

Temporal Lobe Functions

- Memory
- Understanding language (receptive language)
- Sequencing
- Hearing
- Organization

Source: Nucleus Medical Media. (2009). Living *with Brain Injury.* Retrieved June 13, 2012. www.biausa.org/living-with-brain-injury.htm by permission.

I was trying to figure it all out. I was trying to find answers but ultimately I had to go inward for those answers; to connect to God and know that all of this was in His divine order, and that God had a plan. I turned inward to my faith and tried to be grateful for the progress my son had made.

At this point I was more confused than before the parent session. I went back to Orion's room to find him lying there with that blank stare. My glow from the previous hour had faded away, but my memory of our time in the pool remained vivid. We had shared so much joy. I held onto that memory. It would give me strength to survive another day. In fact each night as I closed my eyes, I tried to concentrate on one good thing that had happened that day. Tonight I would remember our time in the pool. Collectively these small steps forward would form the miracle I was hoping and praying for every day.

Once again I realized all my attention was on Orion and I turned my thoughts to my precious son, Noah. How must he feel? He was attending high school and concentrating on graduating soon. Meanwhile, his brother was in some rehab hospital fighting to get his life back. His mom was by his brother's side while his Dad was trying to work and hold the family together. Thank goodness for good friends. Noah had plenty of them and they were there for him. We tried to keep his life as normal as possible, but I know his heart was breaking like the rest of us.

I really wanted to be near him, to hold him, to talk with him and hear how school was going but I had no choice other than to be here with Orion. I knew I was exactly where I needed to be but that did not make it any easier. I still missed Noah dearly and hoped that he would someday understand how much I loved and missed him during this time. When I did call him I tried to sound so strong and hoped he could feel some comfort behind my words. I'd tell him his brother was going to be just fine, but I'm sure he could hear the uncertainty behind my words. I felt I couldn't leave Orion even for a moment. For me, it was like having an infant all over again. Noah would have to switch rolls and become big brother for a while.

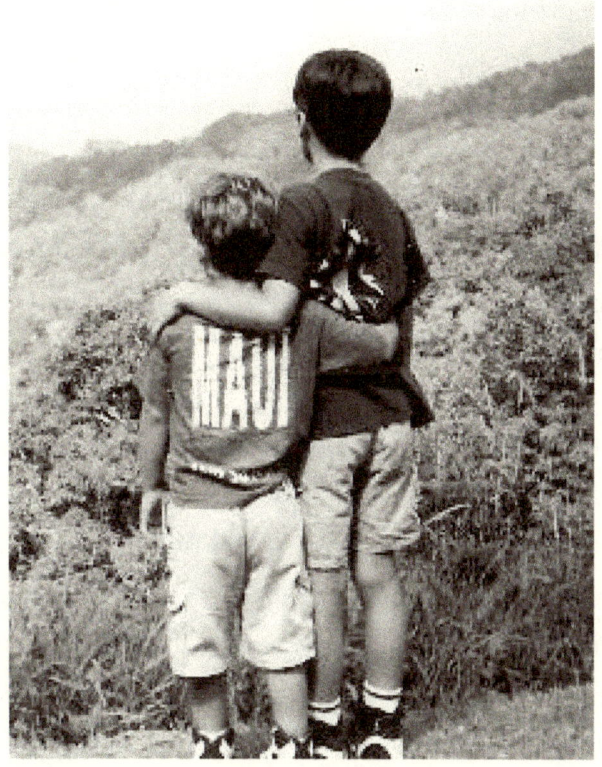

**Noah and Orion looking out at
the mountains while on vacation**

Although my life revolved around Orion's recovery there were times I was forced to address issues outside the rehab facility. For example, my friend Vita had been working very hard to sell some of our homes due to financial reasons. She had an offer on one home and needed both mine and Bill's signatures to close the deal. This would be only the second time I had left Orion, the first being the time we left him to go to the tow truck company.

I told Orion I would be back at 1:30 pm sharp. He looked lost but finally nodded in agreement. I gave him a clock, placed it close by, and told Orion that when this hand is here and here I would be back. I was nervous to leave him but the nursing staff reassured me that he would be just fine. I couldn't believe I felt this way, but I still had such a fear of losing my child.

We met Vita at the reality company. She had all the paperwork ready. It was so good to see her under these circumstances, rather than the last time I had seen her at the hospital. She is a very close friend and I love her dearly. We hugged and I told her how much I appreciated everything she was doing. Then we signed the paperwork, said our goodbyes and left. Thankfully, there did not appear to be a problem getting back to the rehab facility by 1:30 as promised. I had barely processed that thought when we received a call that there was something else to sign. Now I was anxious and the clock was ticking, but my husband reassured me that Orion would be just fine. Nevertheless, I called the facility and the nurse told me that he was doing fine. They had laid him down after therapy and he was sound asleep.

Then, at exactly 1:30, we were still on the expressway and I got a feeling something had happened. It's a gut feeling; an intuition only a mother understands when it comes to her children. It seemed to take forever to get back to the facility.

We arrived at the rehab facility later than promised, at approximately 2:30 pm. As we headed to Orion's room we were stopped by the nurse who informed us that at 1:30, Orion managed to climb over the bed rails and fall. I was really scared as I knew a slight bump on his head could mean more bleeding in his brain, possibly more brain damage or even death. I rushed to his side. Thankfully, he had only a few minor bumps and bruises but otherwise looked fine.

Orion looked right at me and said, "You lied. I was coming to find you Mom." I explained we had gotten tied up with the real estate deal before it dawned on me that he actually knew what time it was. This was huge! I was so relieved that my son knew when 1:30 came!

It was still painful for me to see my once strong, strapping college graduate ready to start his career and life thrown back to start all over again. Thoughts raced through my mind. Would he ever walk? Would he get a job? Or would he get married and have children? Would Orion ever achieve or reach his goal to drive again? All of these questions engulfed the constant chatter of confusion and uncertainty of what lie ahead for my beautiful son. Around each turn of the bumpy, winding road to recovery lie the unknown.

During such difficult moments I would hear the sound of Orion's voice saying, 'Never give up.' He had said this to me one night as the day wound down to a close. I had settled him for the night when he nodded for me to come closer. I looked in his eyes as he whispered, "Mom, I'm here to teach you something." I said, "You're here to teach me? What would that be, son?" He whispered softly, "To never give up – no matter what."

A tear rolled down my cheek as I gazed at his crooked little smile. I held his hand tightly and said, "Son, I'll never give up – ever." He nodded to reassure me that he wouldn't either. I continued "and besides, you are as stubborn as your mother!" He grinned as he dozed off to sleep.

LOVE AND SUPPORT

The nights were long as the uncertainty crept in. I needed my big sister. I needed my family. I needed my friends. I wanted my life back the way it was but I knew it was forever changed. I would call my older sister Debbie because she had a son the same age as Orion. In fact, my younger sister Ronnie, older sister Debbie and I were all pregnant at the same time. All of us had boys the same age. I had lost touch with my other sister Monica, but knew she was praying for Orion's recovery.

Debbie would talk and comfort me as a big sister. She tried to tell me that Orion would be just fine, but I could hear the uncertainty in the tone of her voice. It still eased my mind as I wanted to believe her words more than anything else in the world.

After Orion was tucked safely into bed at night I would call her from the hallway. I needed to hear her voice but also knew as I began to talk the tears would start flowing. I couldn't let Orion see or hear me in this vulnerable state. The halls were bare and sterile as I paced up and down explaining Orion's progress. She had a way of saying just what I needed to hear so I looked forward to hearing her voice after the end of every day. Debbie allowed me to express my fears and expectations and cry uncontrollably without judgment. I love her dearly.

My little sister Ronnie and my mom visited often. I tried to be brave and strong, but Ronnie and I were very close and she knew the pain I was feeling. My mom had always been there for me and it hurt to see the despair and concern on her face. I greatly admire Ray, my stepfather, and knew it was hard for him to visit hospitals. But I also knew he would be there for me any time if I needed a friend, as he always had. I could call on Ray for anything; sometimes even just to vent and tell him how I was feeling. His words were comforting and helped me immensely. He is very special to me.

Bill's sister Rebca also visited often. She has big blue eyes like her mother. After Orion's feeding tube had been removed he was able to eat mostly mashed foods. I had told Rebca the good news. She knew Orion's favorite food was deviled eggs, so she said, "We can mash them and it will be fine." I told Orion that Aunt Rebca was bringing deviled eggs and I could tell he was excited by the look on his face.

The next day Rebca showed up with her famous deviled eggs. Before we could mash anything, Orion grabbed one with his "good' hand and popped the whole thing in his mouth! We both looked shocked as he chewed it up and reached for another. I had to hold him back just a little or he would have eaten the entire dozen on the spot! Once we were sure Orion wasn't going to choke, we hugged each other and then my son. We knew he was well on his way to recovery.

We spent the rest of the day reminiscing about how far Orion had come and sharing memories of past times together. One topic was that of my son telling his aunt that her deviled eggs were much better than his moms. Obviously, he still felt that way!

Bill's brother Robert lived much further away, but he and his wife Diane would take time regularly to send cards to Orion. It seemed as if they mailed one a day as we hung them all around his room. It warmed my heart to see the look on my son's face as he anticipated coming back after a long day to find a new card on his bed. Those cards meant so much to him. I was grateful Robert and Diane set aside time to send them.

One day before Orion's friends Dante, Joey and JT came to visit, I frantically ran to the office supply store located directly across the street from the rehab facility. I needed to make copies of some information I had collected to help them understand Orion's condition. The pages contained such things as symptoms usually associated with TBI and many of the changes they might observe during their visit with Orion such as change of behavior, impulsivity, anger, lack of awareness and so on. I made a folder for each of them because I knew they had no understanding on the subject of brain injury and I thought the information might help them. I handed each of them a folder and explained what I had done. I mentioned that although Orion's injury was on his left side, he had most of the right sided deficits.

Looking back, I think those three kids must have been scared to death. They probably thought I'd gone off the deep end; distributing entire educational packets on brain injury. Thank God these young men love me. I hope they look back and chuckle about my 'temporary insanity'. Meanwhile Orion just stared with a blank look on his face, probably wishing he could express his feelings of embarrassment. The funniest part was when his friend Joey said, "Great Orion, now you come with instructions!" We all laughed and I noticed Orion's smile was getting much better.

Day after day friends and family came to see my son and show their love and support for our family. While I tried to show strength and courage around them, inside I felt as if I was dying. Even though I knew Orion was making huge strides forward, I had become emotionally exhausted. My husband Bill, a very spiritual man and someone I loved dearly, probably suffered my wrath the most. I was hurting inside and my marriage was suffering as a result. I was not sure why. He was doing the best he could, but in my mind I always expected more.

Bill says that during this time he learned the difference between men and women. He was always calculating this or that and I didn't see him being emotionally involved. He believes men hide from their emotions and that 'real men' don't cry. Or do they? I later learned this had affected him as much as me. We were both trying to deal with this devastating event in our own way. Bill feels that many marriages fail during tests of this type because each person is not willing to understand and accept the difference between the way a male and a female deal with trauma and stress. The 'blame game' can easily take hold and can do irrefutable damage to a relationship in this type of situation.

As women we are very emotional and can burst into tears at the slightest little thing. Men, on the other hand, are taught to be tough and to hold it all together at any cost. It didn't seem to matter what Bill did, it wasn't ever good enough, and I wanted more.

I now understand he was doing the best he could at the time but I simply couldn't see it. It's been said we take out our frustrations on the ones we love the most. I certainly did. I was emotionally raw and needed comfort. Even today I don't think anything my husband said or did at the time could have supplied that comfort. I wanted him to *fix* my son and make everything all better.

We were all under so much stress. While Orion and I were going through our grueling routine five days a week, life outside the hospital continued on. My husband and I owned several rental properties and the demands of real life kept coming at us. Escalating bills, unhappy tenants, maintenance of the properties and the demands of everyday life took its toll. I realize now that we were both feeling the pressure coming at us from all directions.

It didn't help that I saw marriages crumbling all around me, including my own. I saw mothers working tirelessly with their children while their husbands were home trying to maintain their job, pay the bills and arrange for the care of other siblings. The men were taking on their own roles as well as many of those traditionally handled by the women.

At the same time each mother's focus was on one thing and one thing only; the child that needed them at that time. There were no words anyone could say to make the pain go away. Looking back I now understand that men and women handle traumatic experiences differently, and I now agree with my husband; we were both hurting in our own ways.

HOMEWARD BOUND

Day after day, week after week, we tried the swallow test but Orion kept failing. The day of discharge drew near. If he couldn't pass the test prior to our departure, we would need to puree his foods and use thickeners in his fluids at home as was being done at the facility. Orion choked and gagged through at least eight to ten swallow tests with no luck. In between testing, I would place an herbal food on his tongue to work his gag reflex.

On the day he was to come home, we were scheduled for one last swallow test. The doctors had written a prescription for a thickener as he could not yet swallow thin liquids. They performed the final test. Lo and behold, he did it! Orion was so excited! Not about passing the test, but that he and his brother could now have a cola! Orion knew that Noah had held up his end of the bargain and he was so excited to share the good news. He immediately took my cell phone, hit his brother's number and said, "You ready for that cola?" I was so happy! Many times it's the simple things in life that bring the most joy. Who would have known the idea of having a cola with his brother could make such a difference. I ripped up the prescription for the thickeners and off we went to prepare for discharge.

I was extremely exhausted at this point; mentally, physically, and most of all emotionally drained. But we were going home! I was relieved to leave the rehab facility and move on to our life at home, but I was also very apprehensive about what lie ahead. For me this was a whole new beginning. What challenges would we face? Only time would tell.

Orion's discharge entailed much more than simply a doctor's signature. There was plenty of preparation that had to be done first. We had to decide upon and purchase a wheelchair and a shower chair along with many other items that would be needed to care for Orion in our home. Thank goodness the therapists were there to help us get ready. They measured the bathrooms for the shower chair, made sure his wheelchair would fit through the doors and offered advice as to how best to get ready for Orion's return home.

I remember watching him sit there in the rehab wheelchair as they measured him for his very own chair. He had specific requirements. The chair must be black and most importantly, the adjustable camber on the wheels. I guess in his mind if he couldn't yet drive a car he would make sure that his wheelchair moved with the highest precision.

Orion had to have a splint made too. It would keep his hand straight while he slept at night. Without the splint his arm would contract and his hand would ball up into a fist before the morning arrived. I had to speak with the doctor so I told the therapist I would meet her afterwards. The therapist was an energetic, young lady and Orion really liked her; it was written all over his face. She would accompany

Orion throughout the procedure and explained the entire process to me before I left to see the doctor. I knew Orion was in good hands. I returned from the doctor consultation to find my son with a fluorescent, hot pink brace! I was shocked and asked, "Of all the colors to choose from son, why hot pink?" He pointed to the therapist and said, "She likes that color mom." And so it was.

Discharge was a bittersweet feeling. Although I was eager to leave the rehab facility, my mind wondered if I would be capable of handling what would come next. Orion still struggled with walking, speech and impulsive behavior. I became overwhelmed as thoughts of our future raced through my mind. As I felt my anxiety begin to rise, I turned to gratitude instead; gratitude that Orion was still here with us. I knew we were so fortunate to be bringing our son home instead of visiting a gravesite.

But Orion was so very different now. The son I raised and loved was no longer there. The new Orion was impulsive, had awareness issues, and physical and cognitive deficits. I realized that I had built up anxiety, confusion and anger inside as to why this had happened to my son. I went through the daily motions on the outside, but my heart had broken to pieces.

I came to the conclusion that I had to hold a private service for the son I had lost. There were no attendees. This one was between me and God. I had to say goodbye to the son that was no longer there and begin the process of getting to know the new guy that was now my child. It may seem strange to some, but I had to find closure so that our new life could begin.

My thoughts were to never give up hope that someday, somehow my son would regain his independence. This was the outcome I longed and prayed for. I would keep moving forward and strive to help my son reach the most important goals; to drive, live independently, and hopefully someday marry the girl of his dreams.

Finally the day had come. We were homeward bound. Orion was now able communicate, dress and feed himself and continued to make strides in the right direction. He was discharged home with outpatient therapy. It would be difficult, but this was the next step in Orion's journey to recovery. He had come a long way and still had a way's to go. Though we were nervous and anxious, our son was coming home just where he belonged. I had prayed so long and hard for this day. Thank you, God!

OUTPATIENT THERAPY

Once Orion was at home, I started looking into outpatient programs. Although we had medical insurance, it did not cover all of the therapies that Orion required. Therefore, money was an issue, so I had to apply for whatever financial aid services I could find to continue his rehabilitation. I was able to locate an outpatient program that accepted him. Although the travel was an hour and a half each way, Bill and I were determined to do whatever we could to help our son overcome his limitations.

Fortunately Bill's sister, Rebca that lived in the same city as the outpatient rehab center. She and her husband kindly offered their spare room for Orion and I to stay through the week. I was very thankful because the long daily drive would have been too difficult for us.

The outpatient program would last four to six weeks, Monday thru Friday 9am-5pm. Weekends we planned to travel home to be with Bill and Noah. My younger son was very happy to have his big brother home. Although my life was still very busy with Orion's activities, I was grateful to see my boys and have weekends with both of them at last.

On the first day of outpatient therapy I realized we were at a new level of Orion's recovery. We arrived at the facility and parked the car. I slung the wheelchair from the back of the truck, brought it around to the front, assisted my son into the chair and off we went for the next leg of our journey.

Once inside the classroom I felt a little out of place. Orion was the only one in a wheelchair and the six to seven other patients seemed 'normal;' no speech deficits, facial droops or no left or right weakness noted. It made me wonder if we had come to the right place. The session began by the instructor going over the day's agenda. Everyone except Orion had an opinion. As he stared off into space I realized I was the only caregiver in the room and I suddenly felt very awkward. How would Orion manage without my assistance? I didn't feel it was safe to leave him alone. Part of his injury was the awareness of his deficits and he had tendency to be very impulsive. In other words, the part of his brain that controlled his awareness was not working. I knew he would try to walk the first chance he got and most likely fall. I couldn't chance it, so I decided to stay.

The patients played a lot of word and memory games during the beginning of the session. As I observed the games, I noticed how the other patients' memories, vision and speech had been affected. Their ages ranged from thirty to sixty years old. Orion was the youngest and obviously the most severe case. Unfortunately, he was unable to participate at this stage. My heart went out to the patients of every age trying to re-gain their lives. They struggled with so many simple tasks. I watched as they focused so hard to find the right word, only to have something completely unrelated pop out of their mouth. I remember the frustrated looks on their faces. Other times they did remember or say the correct word and would smile from ear to ear with joy. I knew it would take time and patience, but I had already seen how far Orion had come and knew inside he would continue to improve. My faith and heart were certain of it.

As part of the therapy, the patients would write down questions and then take turns answering them. I felt Orion was at a huge disadvantage during this exercise. Prior to the accident he was left-handed and his left hand still did not function. I tried to write for him but was stopped as soon as I began. A therapist passed by and placed a pen in Orion's right hand. I explained to her that he was left-handed. She simply stated, "Not anymore." Her comment seemed rude and I could see our personalities didn't work well together.

Orion attempted to scribble his answers with his right hand. It looked like a kindergartner's writing, which made sense because he was learning to write all over again. Meanwhile, I was still frustrated with the therapist. Didn't she know how her actions and words made me feel? She had a young son. How would she like it if her son's entire life had been ripped out from under him? I realized it was my inward questioning to God; my inner struggle that had nothing to do with her, and there was no sense in harboring any anger. My reaction was really the result of my sadness and fears surfacing. I loved my son and he had such wonderful goals and plans. Now here we sat in a room of patients playing simple games he couldn't even understand. It seemed so unfair.

Then my mind went back to the struggle Orion underwent when he tried to dress himself that first day in rehab and when he was learning to feed himself with his right hand. Weeks of practice and his sheer determination allowed him to learn and eventually master these tasks. Writing would be just one more challenge. In fact, if my son was ever going to write again, he would have to do it with the pen in his right hand. I realized the therapist's action was the best thing she could have done.

Sometimes I was allowed to sit and observe the sessions. It was difficult as there was a wide variety of patients. Everyone from professionals to soldiers to students joined Orion in therapy. Most couldn't even find words to say, which is common with TBI patients. I could see the frustration building as they tried to talk sometimes with tears pouring from their eyes. My son had the most apparent physical problems. Some of the patients were doing so well a person would never have known he or she had a brain injury until they heard them speak. It was very encouraging to see them improve from week to week as they strived to recapture their lives.

In between therapy sessions I tried to learn everything I could about brain injury. It is a strange, complicated injury that affects individuals very differently. Through my research I learned the scope of the injury is usually dependent on the area of the brain that was injured. There are two sides of the brain and each hemisphere is responsible for different body functions and skills. In most people, the left side controls the language centers and the right side manages cognitive skills such as attention, memory, organization, reasoning and problem solving. There are areas of the brain designed to control body functions, speech, sight, awareness, impulsivity and personality, to name a few. In Orion's case, multiple areas of the brain were affected. I learned in the early stages of his recovery that the extent of injury, recovery, timeline and details of every person's recovery plan is unique to him or her. No two injuries or recoveries are the same.

I saw Orion run into walls with his wheelchair and sometimes even get lost on his way to the therapy rooms. I had to step back and let the therapists do their job. They were trying to help him regain his independence without mommy stepping in around every corner. I knew he had to learn. Some days I could watch while other days I would find a private place to spend my day crying and asking God "Why?"

Orion's outpatient therapies included cognitive, physical, speech and occupational sessions. Orion was not capable of participating in the cognitive therapy games at this point. He simply sat and stared through the sessions. I wasn't much different as I stared in disbelief. I watched the patients struggle to find their words and perform the requested task. This too got better with time. Eventually, I began to see my son participate and watched in amazement as his performance of the tasks became less complicated.

One day in occupational therapy, the therapist said, "Okay, Orion. Make me a sandwich." By this point Orion could lean on the counter to keep his balance. He pulled out bread, mustard and sliced cheese. The therapist asked, "What about the meat and mayonnaise?" He replied, "I am a vegetarian and I *hate* mayo!" She laughed and said, "Well, cheese sandwich it is."

He proceeded to slab the mustard on the bread. The next step of opening the sliced cheese would be more of a challenge. We tend to take these simple tasks for granted. He removed the wrapper and the cheese fell to the floor. The therapist balanced him as he leaned over, picked it up and placed it on the bread. She asked, "Are you going to put that on the bread after it dropped to the floor?" He replied, "Haven't you heard of the three second rule?" She laughed and continued, "No tomato? No lettuce?" Orion said, "Nope. I like mine with cheese and mustard," as he proceeded to take a bite of his sandwich. My son's personality and sense of humor were coming back! Although he was very different from the son I knew before, he was getting better, and for this I was grateful.

During physical therapy he worked relentlessly on his balance. His left side was still weak but his persistence and determination were strong.

One day the therapist brought him over to the treadmill, strapped him safely to the machine and got him started. Orion did his best while the therapist stepped aside to monitor another patient. He was just about finished when a lady came to use the machine. The therapist stopped the treadmill and Orion struggled to get off. I heard the lady mention to her friend, "We have to wait until the retard gets off." I knew Orion heard her by the look on his face. He had been so happy before and so proud of his walking session. In one moment his face drooped and all hope faded away. I knew if I said anything to the lady I would lose control. If only she knew the depth and destruction behind such a hurtful, unnecessary comment. Since I didn't want to end up having said something I might regret, I channeled my energy to Orion. I encouraged him by telling him how well he had done and that he was making great progress. He was improving more and more each day and I was very proud of him. More importantly, his mind was getting better, along with his physical strength.

Another area of the brain that was affected was Orion's speech. His voice was very flat, monotone and difficult to understand. I sat through speech therapy and listened as he tried different tones, but every note seemed the same. Orion had asked me to wait outside the room during several therapy sessions. I later learned he was preparing something special for me. I gave him his space and anxiously sat outside the door while he practiced his surprise over the course of the next couple of weeks.

One day the speech therapist invited me in. She was a kind and gentle woman with a soft voice. "Today," she began, "We have a surprise for you. Orion has been practicing a Led Zeppelin song and would like to sing it to you." She quietly reached over and put on the background music. Orion faced me with a gleam in his eyes and his only slightly crooked smile and asked, "Ready, Mom?" I said, "You bet." He began to sing in a voice that was music to only a mother's ears. The song was *All My Love* by Led Zeppelin. Although he sang out of tune, it sounded beautifully to me. Tears poured down my cheeks uncontrollably as he bellowed the words to chorus, "All of my love, all of my love, all of my love to you, mom."

I tried to regain my composure, but I was overwhelmed with emotion. Orion's eyes looked straight into mine as he continued to sing the lyrics he had worked so hard to perfect. It was the sweetest music I had ever heard. The song seemed to be bursting out of him! I wanted to jump up and give him a great big hug. Instead, I sat and stared in his sparkling eyes as he sang the entire song.

When he finished, my son reached over with his good hand and said, "That was for you, mom. What do you think?" My voice trembled as I said, "That was amazing! It's the most beautiful song I have ever heard son. Thank you." He flashed a smile and his face lit up as if he had just conquered the world. There was so much love between us. The words 'all of my love to you mom' played over in my mind throughout the day and into the night. The memory of my son singing that song to me remains vivid to this day.

Orion attended outpatient therapies for six weeks. One of the therapies was an occupational therapy, which was used to strengthen his left hand and arm. The main prop for the occupational exercises was a pegboard. He struggled with his weak hand as he concentrated on each challenge. Even if it took a long time he would move the peg. The look of determination on his face was intense as he focused on the development of his left hand coordination.

Orion worked very hard and was making great progress. His willpower and stubbornness was paying off; my son was getting better! As a matter of fact, he had worked so hard that the occupational therapists asked him to demonstrate a device we had purchased to help him recoup fine motor skills in his left hand. Orion was thrilled! He demonstrated the use of the device for some of the therapists that were in training at the time. My sister and mom watched as Orion performed the demonstration with enormous intensity; sweat pouring from his brow. Everyone was very impressed with him and he was so proud. It was written all over his face. We congratulated him on his accomplishment and I thanked each of the therapists for the opportunity they had created for my son.

Orion had come so far and was getting better every day. We had become very close over the course of the last year as he worked to reach his goals. I was his support, while he did all the work. At this point, he could recognize the therapists by name, write with his right hand, feed himself and even his walk had become steadier. My son's smile was beautiful with no drooping of his mouth. All of the hard work was finally paying off! He had even learned to text himself messages on his phone so he could remember things. Orion was moving forward by leaps and bounds. He still struggled with the impulsivity, but I was confident this too would soon improve as his new life continued to unfold.

REGAINING INDEPENDENCE

We were released from the Monday through Friday outpatient therapy routine; however Orion continued to attend therapy sessions less frequently in a nearby town. We had no money to pay for regular therapy sessions, but through the grace of God we were able to continue periodic occupational and physical therapy sessions. I applied for some funding through local organizations so my son could receive the additional help he so desperately needed. Orion went to occupational therapy twice a week to further develop the strength in his arm and hand. There were overlapping physical therapy sessions at the local hospital to exercise his legs and improve his walking stride. In total these additional therapies lasted another six weeks and enabled Orion to move into the next phase of his new life. There are so many amazing moments that come to my mind as I remember my son's difficult road to independence. Here are just a few of the highlights.

COLA AT LAST

I recall an inspirational moment that occurred a few days after we were home. There were my two beautiful sons getting ready to share a cola together, just as they had promised. Although my son's interests were at opposite ends of the spectrum, there is a pact amongst siblings that is in their very nature. My two sons, one loving the surf and the sun while the other preferred the mountains and colder climates, were direct opposites yet they were still brothers and would do anything for one another. They sat across from one another as they raised their cola cans, clunked them together and bottoms up. Of course Orion took a much larger drink than he should have taken. And yes, he gagged and choked a little, but he quickly recovered and went for the next drink. I watched them from a distance to give them their space and relished in the moment. I was overcome with happiness and gratitude. We were all finally together, at home where we belonged.

LAKE AND GYM

Weeks of various therapies had come to an end and all of Orion's hard work had paid off. His physical and mental skills had tremendously improved as he emerged into his new world. Although the formal therapies had ceased, Orion was eager to further build on his physical strength. He and I joined a local gym and went faithfully three days a week. It seemed as though we had reversed roles. Orion was now the one encouraging me saying, "Come on, mom. You can do it!"

He worked out on the machines while I spent most of my time walking a track around a small, tranquil lake. There were beautiful lotus flowers gracefully floating in the middle, and the sound of the birds singing provided background music for the sparkles that danced across the water. As I admired the lotus flowers I compared them to Orion trapped in this body and developing into his new person, just as the lotus bud opens to a stunning flower. I imagined the gold center as Orion's heart surrounded by white petals representing the purity of a new beginning.

Nature's beauty surrounded me as I connected to God in a way that no words can express. I thanked Him for bringing my son back to me and filling me with joy. There was a point in my path where I could see Orion through the glass windows using the exercise machines. He had such a look of determination as he pulled the weights with all his might. I was so proud. Afterward I would join Orion inside. He gave me a hard time as he said, "Come on Mom. You need to work out on the machines too." But I was drawn to the lake. That was where I found my peace.

One day while I was walking, I heard someone running behind me. Most days I would step aside for the occasional jogger passing by. But this day was different. I stepped out of the way and to my amazement, my son went running by. Not walking, but yes indeed, running! His physical limitations inspired his own, perfectly unique gait. It was beautiful. My eyes filled with tears and my heart with gratitude. I had my son back. He was the new and improved version, I said to myself as I giggled with joy. I felt so blessed. Orion was regaining his independence and I finally felt like everything was going to be okay. The smile on his face was so beautiful! To this day, I don't know who was happier, him or me.

MY MOM AND DAD'S ROLES

Shortly thereafter Orion began taking walks with my mom, a petite but strong woman. She took Orion under her wing and the next thing I knew they had become inseparable. She gave him nutritional advice as he listened intently to her every word during their long walks together. Orion quickly became conscious of the environment. As they walked he would pick up cans stating, "I'm going to clean up this place." My mom smiled with pride and approval. They would venture for miles on their walks together, always sure to carry a bag to pick up the trash along the way.

Orion's walks with my mom were therapeutic and enlightening for both parties. He admired my mom, as did I, and listened intently to her advice. She had become Orion's personal fitness trainer and nutritional coach. Mom made healthy soups, smoothies and other good foods for him. She would take time with him at the grocery store to point out the ingredients and nutritional content on the labels. Orion soaked up the new found knowledge. As she told the story, my mind drifted back to the time my son could not even locate the bright, yellow bag of M&M's and now he was reading labels. He had come such a long way.

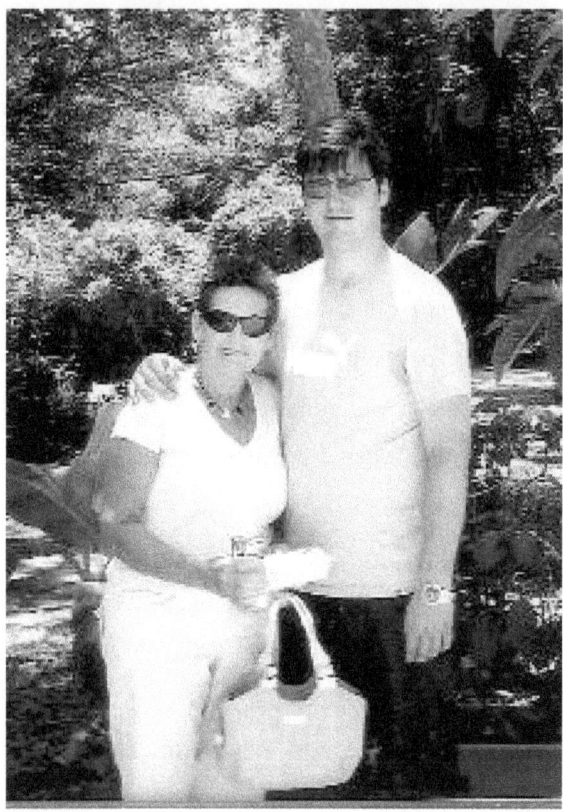

Orion and my mom

Orion also loved to rave about how my mom was such a good cook. Our family had a long-standing joke that my cooking was not quite up to par, so Orion took every opportunity to point that out. I didn't take offense to his comments; cooking was simply not my best attribute and I was appreciative my mom took the time to advise and teach him healthy eating habits.

I was grateful the two of them had become very close as I was mentally and physically drained from the nearly fifteen months of constant care for my son. I knew it was time for me to step back and let my mom take over while I reunited with Noah and my husband. I watched in amazement from a distance as Orion and my mom established a remarkable bond; one that I thought only possible between a mother and her child. He often teased, "I have two moms," and I would reply, "No son, I am your one and only, but I will share." He grinned and we hugged each other. Although the time had come for me to step back, our closeness had become infinite and beyond words.

My mom was very health conscious and it showed. In the weeks and months that followed, the two of them became very close. She joined the gym where Orion worked out. They went together, separated to do their own workouts and got back together for a walk at the end of their session. Their bond and love for one another continues to grow to this day.

Recently my mom and I discussed the relationship between the two of them. I wanted her to know how much I appreciate all she does for Orion. She smiled and started reminiscing about some of their past walks and special times together. She mentioned a time when Orion was in his recycling mode. They had walked along a long, winding trail that led to the intra coastal waterway. She was admiring some birds on the other side of the water when she turned around just as

Orion climbed over the railing. He was heading for a shiny object dangling in a shrub. It was a can. Her first reaction was that of fear but she was well aware of Orion's determination. Before she knew it he had grabbed the can, made his way back to the edge, pulled himself back over the railing and stood in front of her grinning from ear to ear about his accomplishment. Mom merely opened the bag so Orion could drop the can in with the others and off they went.

She spoke of another time when they had walked around the lake at the gym. There were a few small alligators in the lake they had seen bob their heads up from time to time, only to disappear as they sank back underwater; a common sight for Florida natives. On this particular day she recalled Orion unexpectedly took off running and looked back and as if to say 'step it up old lady.' Unintentionally he was creeping closer to the water's edge each time he looked back at her. He was so intent and focused on his running that when mom mentioned that he was getting a little too close for comfort, he denied it. This type of awareness issue is common in TBI patients. Orion literally didn't realize he could fall in lake if he wasn't careful.

She recalled another similar occasion where Orion made her nervous as well. The two of them were walking along a path when he suddenly said, "Oh come on, let's take this path." It was a treacherous path certainly much more dangerous than the sidewalk they had been on but there was no talking Orion out of his decision. He said, "You can do it." Never once did he question his abilities. His only concern was whether or not my mom would be able to follow his lead.

Impulsivity is something Orion is still dealing with today. She mentioned another occurrence when Orion sped off once again. This time he raced up a hill; thankfully a small one. They made it to the top but on the way back down he was going too fast. He fell down and slid all the way to the bottom of the hill on his bottom. He looked up, smiled at her and said, "I told you we could do it." They laughed and hugged and continued on their journey.

I was constantly afraid of Orion falling and felt such anxiety as my mom told the stories. I knew I had to let him live his life so I prayed that God would watch over him. Orion's determination far surpassed anything that I could ever anticipate. It is what kept him going and continues to do so to this day.

I am so thankful my mom stepped in when Orion was trying to detach from me. My son wanted his independence and that's what I wanted for him. While I stepped back, my mom stepped forward. Orion continues to visit with my mom and stepdad every week. My mom prepares nutritious snacks and he and Ray hang out in their oversized garage talking 'guy stuff.'

I can call on Ray for anything as well as talk to him about anything; sometimes even just to vent and tell him how I was feeling. His words of wisdom were comforting and helped me immensely. He took Orion under his wing when he was trying to regain independence. Ray stepped right up and Orion knew he could ask him anything too. Orion has a lot of respect for him, as do I. I am grateful to have two such caring parents.

eBay Car Story

Orion wanted a car so bad. A few months after we had come home, he was learning how to use his right hand to type. I had given him full access to the keyboard and thought this to be a type of therapy in and of itself. I tried to give him his privacy and refrain from watching over his shoulder. At the same time I needed to make sure he was staying away from unsafe websites and not doing anything that could cause problems.

One day I noticed he was on eBay. Oh my! He was bidding on an extremely expensive car! I panicked and quickly went to get my husband to find out how we could get out of this mess. Orion didn't understand why I was so upset or why he wasn't allowed to buy a car. He simply admired the car and wanted to buy it. Bill and I watched intently as the bidding end drew near. Fortunately one of those last minute bids came through with only seconds left on the clock. My husband and I wiped the sweat from our brows and wondered how we were going to explain the severity of this event to our son. It was difficult because he didn't understand the value of money.

He suffered from another condition common in TBI patients called perseveration. It is the repetition of a particular response, such as a word, phrase, or gesture, despite the absence or cessation of a stimulus. If an issue has been fully explored and discussed to a point of resolution, it is not uncommon for something to trigger the reinvestigation of the matter. This can happen at any time during a conversation. This meant from this day forward he may try to repeat this episode. We could see Orion's new life was going to be quite a challenge for us too.

22ND BIRTHDAY

More than a year had passed since Orion's accident as his twenty-second birthday grew near. Our family wanted to do something special for him to celebrate the event so we planned a twenty-first birthday party. After all, last year we had spent his birthday grateful to have Orion with us as he lay in a coma in the hospital. Yes, a celebration was definitely in order. Orion said, "This is going to be big, mom. I have a lot of time to make up. We can celebrate two birthdays for the price of one!" And so we did.

All of his friends attended. We made a fire in the fire pit. The 'kids' were all grown men now, some with their girlfriends. They laughed and shared memories, past and present. Orion was in his element at last. I remember peering out my window around midnight, before I dozed off to sleep. There were still about twelve friends remaining, including Orion, giggling and reminiscing. I thought, "I will sleep soundly tonight," as the music of their laughter rang in my ears. My heart was full of love and gratitude. Indeed, with God all things *are* possible!

SCREENPLAY

None of us were sure whether or not Orion had determined he would not be able to do his previous job as a camera man, or if perhaps he had switched interests. All we knew was that he had learned to type very fast with his right hand and had begun to write a screenplay. It was titled *Round 2* and was a story about recovery from his perspective.

I didn't get a chance to read it all because Orion wasn't too keen about having mom read his material. As I recall the beginning of the story describes a self-centered college graduate pursuing his career. He goes on to talk about the person he became following the accident. The story explained how his personality had changed; that he became caring and considerate of others. It goes on to describe how he found the inner-strength to make it to where he is today. I was intrigued as I read about recovery from the patient's viewpoint.

Although Orion's story was far different from my caregiver's recollection, both were equally important and informative. Orion's drive and determination within the story was as incredible as it had been throughout his recovery. I was excited at the possibility to share both sides of the coin; his perspective as well as mine. It's 'no accident' that we are both documenting our experience. Each of us, in our own way, seemed to be planning to communicate our story. Each of us wanted to share our experience to offer hope to another person along their journey. It was exciting to me that we might have the opportunity to share with others our experience and perhaps make their situation a little less difficult.

BIKE

Orion had a bike he was eager to ride. Just like training a child, he put on his helmet and pads, I gave him a push and off he went. It was difficult for him because his left leg didn't always cooperate with the pedals. As he got better he would take off on his own. It was hard to watch, but a necessary step towards his independence.

One day as I looked out my bedroom window I saw him attempt to get on his bike. He wore his helmet and bright yellow jacket when riding his new bike. As he tried to sit on it he lost his balance and over he went. His left side did not move and just folded behind him. My first instinct was to run and protect him, but I knew he would be embarrassed and he needed to learn this for himself. I swallowed my pride, wiped away my tears, and continued to watch.

Once again he attempted to get on his bike with the same result, over he went. The saying goes; 'the third time's the charm.' Orion made his third attempt and he made it! He was on the bike and riding down the street as if nothing had happened. It was hard to watch him ride away, but I knew this was an example of what he had worked so hard for over the past two years.

Orion began riding his bike almost daily and became better and better. One day as I was watching him ride away, I remembered what my spiritual teacher, Grace, had said about a vision she had during meditation two years earlier, as my son lay lifeless in the hospital. She said, "I see him on a bike." Her vision had become reality.

ORION GIVES SPEECHES AT REHAB

About two and a half years after Orion's accident, I found myself back in those same rooms of the rehab hospital under completely different circumstances. I recognized the distress and fear on the faces of the mothers in the room. It was a reflection from my own mirror years before.

Today Orion stood proudly in front of those mothers speaking of hope, determination and strength. Today I admired my son, sharply dressed in a beautiful suit and tie he put on by himself. He had a gleam in his eyes and smile on his face as the mothers in the room looked back at him with a spark of hope in their eyes. Orion stood before them as a living example that anything is possible. The theme of his story encouraged them to never give up. As I gazed around the room and saw a glimmer of hope in the mother's eyes, I was so proud of my son and also relieved to be on this end of the long journey. It made me very happy to see that Orion had encouraged the patient's mothers. He made it a little easier for them to get through the days ahead.

About six months later Orion and I sat at the doctor's office awaiting a routine checkup when a mother approached me. She said, "I know you. I was in the room when your son gave that speech at rehab." She proceeded to tell me that her son had a TBI as a result of a car accident. His newborn baby had died in his arms and he was depressed and given up on life. He was in the room that day for Orion's speech. The mother said that after the speech, something snapped in her son. Her eyes filled with tears as she described her son's personal tragedy and she explained that after he heard Orion speak, he started to live again. He began getting up early and trying harder in his therapy sessions. He actually wanted to live! Her eyes filled with tears as the words flowed from her lips. She thanked me over and over and said that Orion was the inspiration who had given her son a second chance at life. I hugged her and our souls connected for just a moment, as if to say, "It's okay. It's going to be okay."

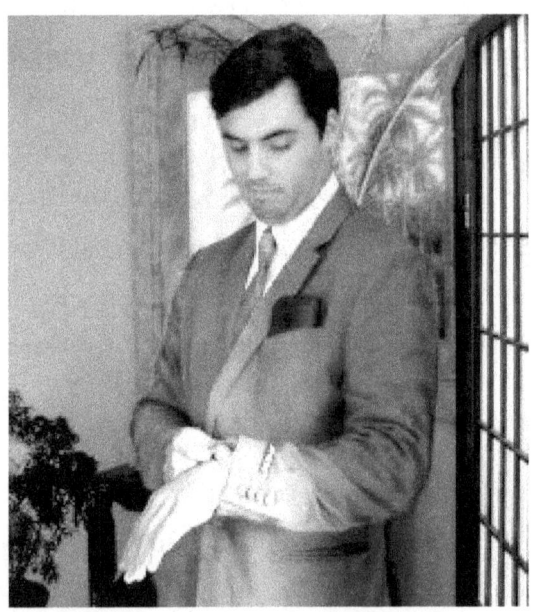

Orion's homage to 'You Only Live Twice'

ORION'S GOAL: DRIVING

Outpatient therapy had lasted about five to six weeks and was now complete. What next? The therapies had ended, the money had run out and now it was up to us to help Orion achieve his most important goal which was to drive again. Once he could drive, we would move on to the dream Bill and I had for our son; to regain his independence. Orion's goal of driving would get him one step closer to our dream becoming a reality.

Fortunately, a new subdivision was being built near our home. In the afternoons, after the construction workers had gone home, my husband would take Orion to the empty lot and put him behind the wheel. He said the grin on his face was huge! In Orion's mind, he thought he was doing great behind the wheel. In reality he couldn't do five MPH and keep the car in a steady line. He would weave from one side of the road to the other.

Nonetheless, Bill would take him out almost daily to practice. My husband would come home and tell me how scary the lesson was. Bill was concerned that maybe he shouldn't be encouraging him to practice. But my husband would not let his son down. Driving really seemed to be Orion's sole purpose and it was the goal that had kept him going for so long. His dream of driving again had been the force of determination behind so many of his accomplishments.

It would take many months for Orion to begin to learn basic driving skills. I emphasize 'begin,' as it would take many more months of practice to master the basic skills needed to drive on the road. But the more he practiced, the better he became.

It had been fourteen months since the accident and Orion was now ready for a driving specialist familiar with TBI to evaluate his skills. The specialist would determine if it was possible for our son to drive again. We contacted a professional in the area and the adventure was underway. Orion spent ten hours with the specialist, each session lasting one to two hours in length. She worked with him to improve braking reaction time, attention, processing speed and insight. The training occurred over a six-month timeframe. With each session Orion hoped he would be released for independent driving even though there was a possibility he might never be able to drive independently again.

During this time his dad and I had permission to continue practice at home. We took every opportunity to take him to undeveloped subdivision for several hours of practice. There were noticeable improvements with every session. We were hopeful our son would reach the goal that the majority had deemed impossible.

After six months, ten hours of professional training and many hours of practice at home, we were on our way to hear the final verdict. Had Orion accomplished his long awaited goal? We sat anxiously awaiting the results.

The therapist arrived and explained how far Orion had come. Unfortunately, she then proceeded to tell us that although Orion had made remarkable improvements, he would still require parental supervision to drive. He was now two years post injury and his recovery was nothing short of miraculous. We weren't about to surrender to this battle! Fortunately, neither was the specialist. She made several recommendations and indicated Orion would be ready for reevaluation in four to six months. He was to continue to practice with parental supervision as long as we had his doctor's permission, and he did not drive on interstates or at night.

Although the look on Orion's face was that of disappointment, I believed there was hope that his dream would someday come true! Two years ago we were praying he would make it through the night and today we are sitting in a driving evaluation meeting! I spent the next two hours driving home with my son telling him how proud I was of him and how we would simply practice that much more and try again. And that is just what we did; every chance, every opportunity, we drove. This had become our new mission.

After months of additional practice it was time for re-evaluation. This time, another driving specialist took him for a spin, and made a few suggestions, including special mirrors and a spinner knob for the steering wheel. Over the past few months, Orion had repeated over and over that if he couldn't drive, it would be the end of the world to him. We tried to tell our son otherwise, but to Orion achieving this goal was everything. In my mind, I kept repeating, "With God all things are possible". After all, look how far he had come. My mind drifted back to nearly two years prior when my son was rapidly pointing to the word 'driving' on the letter board. Indeed, he would drive again. We just needed to keep pushing forward.

Finally, we heard the words we were praying to hear, "I see no reason why this young man cannot achieve his goal." These words were music to our ears. Orion lit up like a child at Christmas. His eyes sparkled and he smiled from ear to ear. Orion was well on his way to achieving his goal and we would do anything to support him along the way.

The new driving specialist had given hope. Orion continued to practice and we made the adjustments to our car as suggested. We would drive one and a half to two hours once or twice a month for ongoing professional training. It went well and Orion was making remarkable progress. He faithfully worked on the specialist's suggestions and practiced daily.

As I look back, I can still hear my son's voice on that lonely dark night two and a half years before saying, "Never give up, mom." And we never did. We kept moving forward, leaving the past behind us, where it belongs. We had hope, faith and strength with us as we watched our son reach towards new goals. It is said, 'The sky's the limit." Each day he reached for the stars!

Orion's driving sessions were over and once again we found ourselves anticipating the outcome of the instructor's evaluation. Would today be the day? We sat in anticipation. Finally the specialist came into the room and gave us the news. Orion was capable of independent driving with a few restrictions. His dream had become a reality! One more miracle had unfolded before us. Orion gleamed! My mind drifted back to the day he set his goal. I could see my son in his hospital bed, unable to speak, as he spelled the word 'drive' on the letter board. And now, almost three years later, it had come to pass. Never – and I mean NEVER give up! Anything is possible!

Although Bill and I had strived for our son to reach his goal, reality soon set in and we realized Orion would be getting behind the wheel and driving away on his own. "Mom, I'm heading to the gym," he would say as he passed us on his way to his car. I watched out the window and felt the fear and anxiety start to take hold. But just as quickly I snapped out of it. This was the day I had waited for and now it was here. I would once again rely on my faith in God and express my gratitude to Him for another miraculous action. My faith had kept me going all along, and today was no different. I smiled and waved to my son as I watched him adjust his mirrors, buckle up and pull away. The grin on his face was from ear to ear!

As time passed, it got easier to watch him head out to the gym, grocery store or visit with family or friends. He was now an independent young man; buying groceries, driving a car, working out at the gym and visiting friends. His new life was unfolding before our eyes just like the 'good old days' before this journey began. Thank you, God.

CALIFORNIA

Orion set many goals. One of them was to visit his friends in California. He had longed for the visit and my husband and I had to come to terms with the fact that somehow we had to let him go. We wanted so much for our son to live a life of normalcy. However this was not an easy task. Even as a young child we had sheltered he and his brother, fearful they would get hurt or even worse, the very real fear of losing them.

We didn't let Orion know we had so much anxiety about his anticipated trip to California. Of course, my thoughts raced with questions like, "What if he misses the plane or doesn't catch his connecting flight? What if he can't read the small print? What if he doesn't recognize his friends? What if his friends don't show up, or they get tied up in traffic?"

In the meantime Orion was excited and feverishly planning his trip. This would be the first time he would be away from his parents for any length of time since the accident. We couldn't let him down. I wanted to help him pack his clothes all nice and tidy. Instead he grabbed his favorite crumpled tee shirt and threw it in the suitcase. He packed the remainder of his bag, refusing any help from me. I had to remind myself this was his trip, not mine. That was easier said than done.

As Bill drove us to the airport, I was going crazy with anxiety, but tried desperately not to show it to Orion. We arrived and walked our son to the security checkpoint where we said our goodbyes. Security asked Orion to empty his pockets, remove his shoes and place them in the basket. To most people, this is simply an inconvenience, but for Orion it took much time and effort. Bill and I watched through the glass as he accomplished one segment of his mission and turned to glance back at us and with a grin before he disappeared into the crowd.

Four hours later my phone beeped, Orion sent me a text message that read, "The eagle has landed!" A text was all I received that trip because he had told me he wouldn't call and I needed to trust him. And that's just what I did. One week later as he exited the plane my heart was full of joy. He had accomplished his mission and returned home safely. This was yet another huge step forward on his journey.

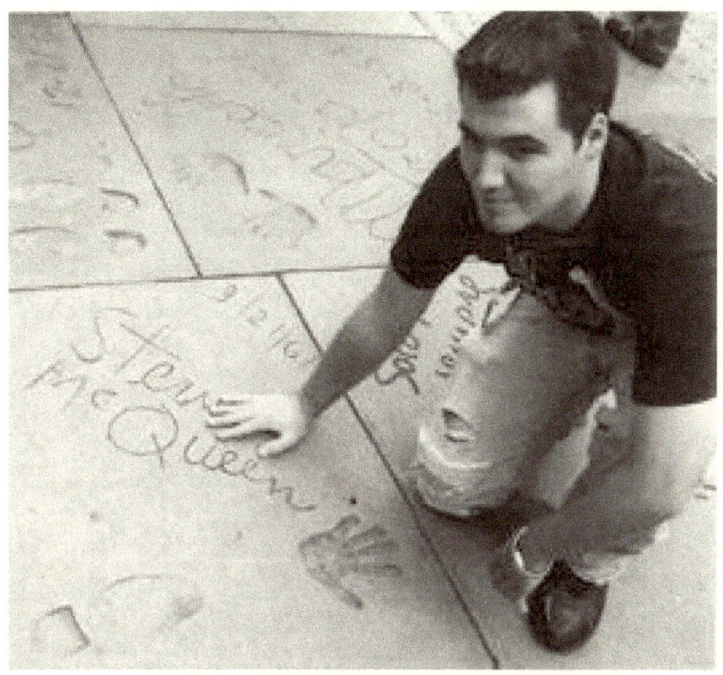

Photo of Orion in California taken by Jon Joy

COSTA RICA POOL STORY

Our family had been through a lot and now we were going to take a break from all the hustle and bustle of therapies and doctors appointments. We decided some much needed time together as a family was in order. I was looking forward to time with my husband and my boys; just the four of us. We planned a trip to Costa Rica. Orion and I planned to leave after a week to get home for some scheduled appointments while Bill and Noah stayed an extra week to enjoy their passion: Surfing. I welcomed any time together with the ones I loved so very much.

I remember one afternoon in Costa Rica as Noah and Bill enjoyed the surf I sat quietly reading a good book and catching up on some much needed R&R. Orion had been taking a nap when I looked up and saw him heading down the stairwell. We were on the second floor at a friend's hotel on the beach and on the ground level was a swimming pool.

I watched as my son walked over to the pool and then, splash, right into the deep end he went! My heart sank. I ran to the bottom of the stairs. My first instinct was to jump in and save him. Instead, I patiently watched as his left arm began to move. He managed his way to the shallow end and looked up at me with that precious smile. I smiled back at him, amazed that he actually did it! I realized nothing was impossible for this young man. He could accomplish anything he set his mind to!

TARIK

As time passed, Orion's friends came and went. Some moved away to begin their own life's journey. Thankfully, Orion's oldest friend Tarik had moved back into town. To Orion's delight, they spent hours together making popcorn, watching movies, and reminiscing about childhood adventures. The two of them were very close friends. I noticed Tarik treated Orion the same as before the accident. Sometimes people tend to talk down to others with a TBI or approach them differently. In reality they want to be treated like they always have been. I appreciated Tarik and the friendship he shared with Orion. He played a vital role in my son's recovery and I am grateful.

One day I walked in the house to hear Orion yell down the stairwell, "Quiet on the set!" I quietly climbed up the stairs and there was my son, dressed in a suit and tie, talking about a research project that he had begun work on. Tarik was behind the camera patiently taping the event as Orion would say, "Take four" or "Take five". On and on he went, striving for nothing less than perfection. That was my son, and I couldn't be more proud.

I admire all of Orion's friends who have stood by him and encouraged him along his journey. Their friendship has helped my son improve at a rapid pace. And Tarik has been a truly dedicated friend. As time passes, Tarik and Orion continue to become even closer.

50TH BIRTHDAY PARTY

On my 50th birthday I had planned to spend a quiet evening at home. Orion, however, would have no part of that! He told me he was going to spend a quiet night at his grandmother's house and he wanted me to go. When my husband and I walked in, I saw all my local family and it was a very pleasant surprise. My little sister and her family, my mom and dad, Noah, and Pop were all there. To my surprise, my sister from Kentucky, Debbie and her husband entered the room. I was shocked! She said, "Thank God you finally made it! Orion had my husband and I trapped in the closet for over an hour, waiting for you!"

Little did I know Orion had been planning the whole event for months and he pulled it off without a hitch! What a wonderful surprise and a loving gesture. Professionals say people with brain injuries have trouble with planning and organizing skills, but this surely wasn't the case with my son! Thanks to him I spent my 50th birthday with my two wonderful sons and all of my loved ones; a good time was had by all!

DRY CLEANER STORY

Orion always parked far away. This habit was something that had been incorporated early on as part of his physical therapy and exercise program. One particular day Orion was on his way to a very important appointment when he pulled up to the local dry cleaners. He parked in the handicap space for the first time ever and ran in to return some hangers. There was an older female customer who commented to the lady behind the counter, "I wish there was a cop around to give that young kid a ticket. Kids just think they can get away with parking in the handicap space." The lady behind the counter looked at her in disbelief, knowing the history of my son. But before she could say anything, the boss and owner of the store came from the back and said, "Excuse me, ma'am. That young man has earned the right to park in the handicap spot. For your information, he is disabled." The lady stood quietly in disbelief and did not utter another word.

At first when I heard what this lady had said, I was very angry inside. I reflected back on the incident that occurred on the treadmill in therapy. Both of these incidents brought about a feeling of sadness. However this time was different. I found myself feeling elation and overwhelming joy. This is because it had been nearly five years from that fateful day and this lady had no idea that my son was even handicapped! She couldn't tell! How great is that?

The moral of the story is don't judge others when you don't know the bumps they have encountered as they make their way down their own winding road to where they are today.

ORION AND POP

Orion and Pop have always been very close but now their bond has grown even closer than before. Orion cares so much for Pop and vise versa. Orion began to take Pop on daily walks. As I watched the two of them out the window as they walked down the street and headed for the beach my heart was filled with happiness and joy.

Pop is now 90 years old and Orion is gentle and patient with him. I watch in amazement as my son cares for his grandfather with such love, kindness and patience. Usually a young man of his age would be into himself but something amazing has happened to my son. He is so caring and compassionate, always going out of his way to help others. He takes Pop out to dinner once a week and dedicates time to visit and take him on walks. Pop looks forward to spending time with him.

As I gaze in amazement at the two of them and see their connection with one another, I am so filled with love and gratitude. I guess when he made the statement as he lay in that rehab bed, barely able to speak, 'mom I'm here to teach you something,' my son truly has taught me a lesson in patience. And he is still teaching me new lessons every day. He takes the time to visit with an elderly neighbor every Sunday, continues to make a point to spend time with his grandparents, and is so loving and patient with others. I think we could all learn a thing or two from his example. I am so proud of him!

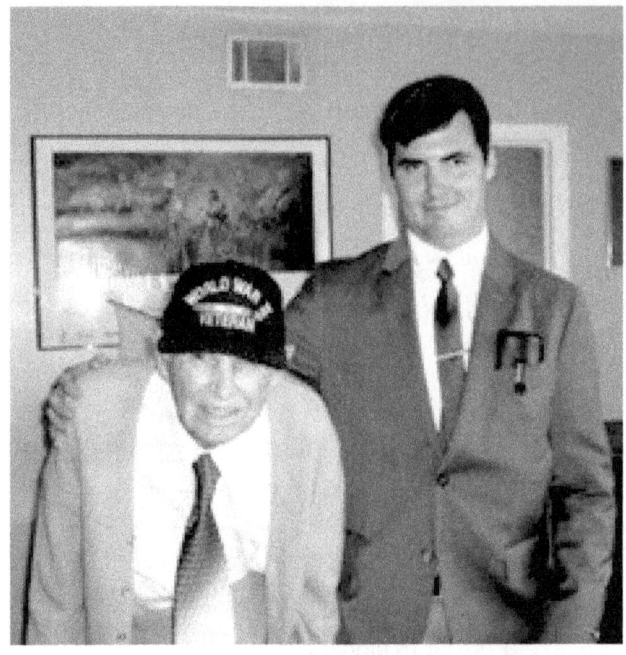

Orion and Pop
James W. Christy gently passed on April 29, 2012.

BAMBOO PLANT

It has always been a big joke between my husband and me that, like my cooking, I do not have a green thumb either. He would make comments like, "You look at a plant and it wilts." Obviously, this is just not my area of expertise. I joke back, saying, "Oh, good! That's one more thing I don't have to do. It's officially your job to water and care for the plants."

I reflect back on a day in the hospital when Grace, my spiritual teacher, gave me a small bamboo plant. She told me to place this in Orion's room in the southwest corner, to look at it every day and say, "Orion, you will grow out of this." And that's what I did. This plant is different because it has meaning. The bamboo plant has sprouted a new branch each significant year of Orion's recovery. There are now three branches and it continues to grow at an astonishing pace.

Our thoughts are very powerful and at the start of each day I look at the little plant and say, "Orion, you will grow out of this." I repeat these words again at the close of each day. Orion, you are still growing out of this. I see it. I feel it. I know it. I believe it. Keep growing to the stars, son! The sky is the limit!

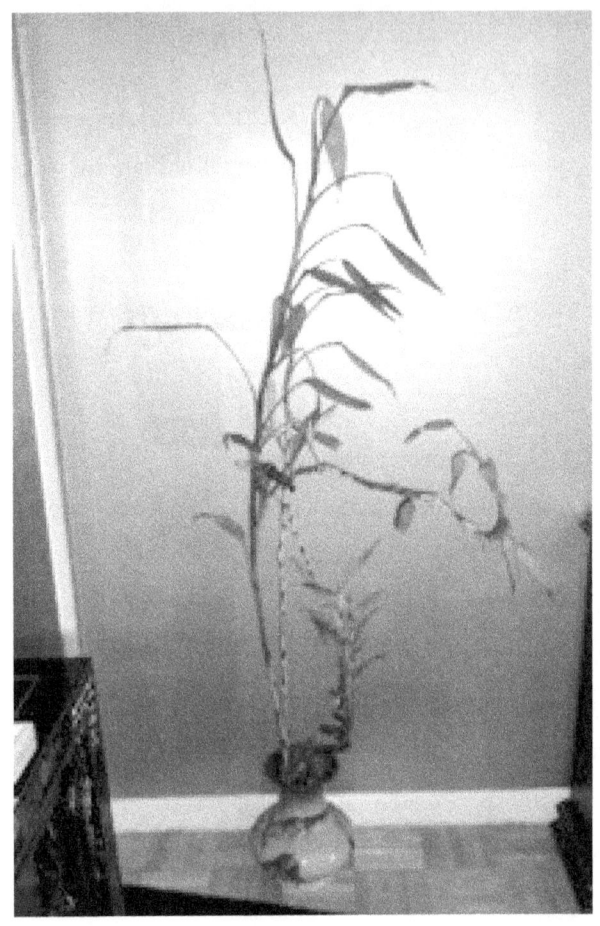

The Bamboo Plant

FAITH AND GRATITUDE

As I look back on Orion's long journey I can't help but wonder. What would have happened if I had listened to the prognosis and the doctors as they told me that my son would be, in their words, 'a vegetable?' Or what if I had placed him in a nursing home like they had originally suggested? What if I had given up and accepted their prognosis as fact? Where would Orion be today?

Although I will never know the answers to these questions, there is one thing I do know. It is that I am so very grateful God took my hand that fateful day and walked by my side throughout my son's journey to recovery. I am grateful for His miracles and His strength and His messages that led me out of the tragic situation.

I continue to rely on my faith that life is all in divine order. As an example, it is *No Accident* that I am writing this book and it is *No Accident* that it is in your hands at this very moment. You see, I believe God has a plan for each of us.

Now as I go through my days I practice meditation, attend Kundalini yoga classes for healing, spend as much time as possible with my children, friends and loved ones and try to never miss an opportunity to tell someone how much I love them. I know far too well how precious life is and do my best to handle life's challenges with Love and Grace, one day at a time.

I reflect on the time that has passed since Orion's accident and realize it's been nearly six years. It all seems surreal. It's like a dream that never happened. Today I sit across the table from my son at his favorite restaurant and watch in amazement as he manhandles a burrito the size of Texas, coated with extra hot sauce. There was a time when we were told that he would always need to take small bites and be careful with swallowing for the rest of his life. Suddenly, I sense the smile on my face and the warmth in my heart as I am overcome with gratitude.

Orion is now living on his own and working on becoming a writer, journalist, and producer. He now drives himself to and from his appointments and still goes to the gym three days a week. I see him walking around town with his new little dog, Claire, and over the causeway bridge, riding his bike, hanging out with friends and going to the movies. He is attending classes for journalism and is writing for an online publication about music, and of course, his other passion; cars. You can visit his website, www.orionchristy.com for more information. He is truly living his life. I had asked God to bring my son back to me and that he did!

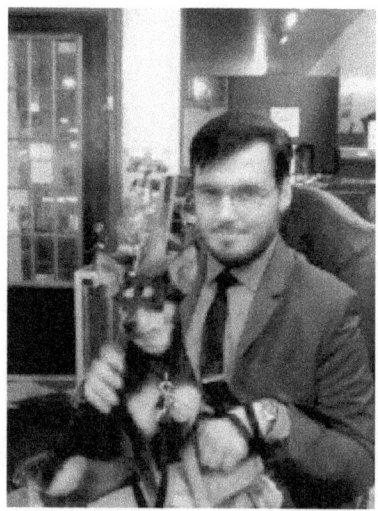

ORION AND A PAL

YOU ARE NOT ALONE

As noted in the previous chapters,
TBI currently affects 1.7 million Americas annually.

5.3 million Americans live with long-term disability
as a result of TBI.

Those of us who have been challenged with TBI stand together and lean on each other. It is a life altering event that leaves every family member, sibling, friend, and patient alike in their own state of uncertainty as to what lies ahead. Anyone who is confronted with a devastating injury or life changing event such as this may find they are unable to think clearly and/or feel as if they simply exist all alone in a world that lies in pieces. That is so far from the truth. We are *not* alone. There *are* ways of seeking and getting help. It is critical to our recovery that we find a place where we can speak about the hurt feelings, anger, shame, resentment, guilt, whatever the case may be, and not be afraid to explore and express our innermost thoughts and feelings.

At times like this we all need to call on family and friends, support groups, therapist, priest, rabbi, pastor or monk, whatever feels right for you. There is no wrong choice. Support systems, in whatever form meets your needs, are there to help us work through the grieving process and the loss of what was a perfect life that is now turned upside down. Keep in mind that a further sense of loss and deeper depression is likely if you try and go it alone. Do not be ashamed to ask for help. Allowing others to help is the first step in healing your aching heart.

Trust me; I understand how difficult it is to take the first step. I was always the type of person that never asked for help and thought I could handle everything all by myself. I came to realize that this time was different. I felt as if I carried the weight of the world on my shoulders, which I later discovered was not only impractical, but impossible. I was hurting inside and had been trying very hard to ignore it, but the sadness just wouldn't go away. It felt like it was embedded deep within my being, on a cellular level. I understood that my son was alive and getting better, yet I was still completely overwhelmed and in a state of despair. What I did not realize was that I had been so busy caring for him that I had not thought about looking at how this life changing event had affected me personally. Yet I kept trying to convince myself that I could handle it.

I had never attended any type of support group or any other program for that matter. But for the sake of my mental and physical health, I finally let go of my ego and attitude of 'I can do it all'. I acted upon the suggestion of a close friend and attended a support group where I found a safe environment around supportive people. They were there to listen and not judge as I worked my way through the pain. This didn't happen right away of course. My difficult journey was filled with buckets of tears, sleepless nights, and countless prayers. It would be weeks before I would find my voice.

Life changing events like this are BIG, so you *will* need help and support as you make your way through your own situation. At times, you may feel isolated or all alone, and think there is no one else who understands your pain. Do not let your mind play tricks on you. This is not true. There are plenty of people who care and programs out there to help. Allow yourself to be open to every option. Do your best to gracefully accept the help of a friend or family member and listen to your heart and try not to judge programs by their label.

Through this experience, I had to let go of the way that *I* thought things should be and trust in my inner intuition to guide me. It's that inner voice that you hear when you learn to quiet your mind from its constant, useless chatter and connect on the heart level to your Source. I learned not only to listen to my inner voice, but to also trust in it. Now when my mind gets in the way, I listen to that inner voice within my heart and know I cannot go wrong.

I found my support program when I asked God to show me the way. And that He did. This occurred when I came to the realization that I couldn't go it alone. I began to trust my inner voice and His guidance. When I did that and let go, magically, I was *led* along my journey. God took my hand and walked by my side. We are never alone.

DEALING WITH OUR GRIEF

If you find yourself feeling overwhelmed, or in the dark depths of despair, please remember that you are not alone in your situation. The fact is that your life, regardless of your relationship to the patient, has been forever altered. You've been traumatized and must allow yourself to journey through a grieving process to get to the 'other side'. As mentioned in the early chapters of this book, I had to learn to let go or say goodbye to my 'old life' so I could begin the process of living my 'new one'.

When we are grieving a real or threatened loss, our self esteem takes a dive. While grieving we may not know the sadness and loss that we feel is only temporary. We tend to lose sight of the 'light at the end of the tunnel' and fear we are doomed to a dark, dreary life of sadness.

There may be times during this traumatic experience that we find ourselves looking for ways to block out all the pain we are feeling. I beg you to seek out healthy alternatives. Create a contact list of individuals, friends, family support groups and keep it with you at all times. I have included many references in the Resources section of the book and the internet offers countless more. We are all vulnerable when faced with extremely painful circumstances that surround TBI. I turned to God, friends, and family and support groups to help me through the dark days.

Grief does indeed take over our lives, so we must be willing to take a risk and seek help from supportive individuals. Our support system persons boost our self esteem through their positive reinforcement. They are the cheerleaders that keep us going when we have no idea how we're going to get through our situation. They help us to realize our strength and we begin to believe in ourselves again. This process of sharing is one of the most helpful and practical ways of working through our grief.

There may be times when we need someone to hold and coddle us, rescue us or tell us to simply 'let time run its course.' As human beings, we need someone to lean on now and then, but remember we are better served when we allow our support persons to simply be there to listen and give us that little nudge when we need it to continue down our path of healing. Embrace their reinforcement, but rely on your own inner strength and perseverance.

I have a particular group of friends that I have met along my journey. I refer to them as 'My Tribe.' This group consists of six wonderful women from all walks of life that God has placed together, to learn, love and grow with each other. I can pick up the phone and I know any one of them would be there for me, as I am for them. It's such a comfort knowing that I don't have to go it alone.

I now know I can count on my supportive groups, spiritual sisters, 'tribal sisters', loving family and friends. They all play their own vital roles in my life. I no longer live in isolation and fear, nor should you.

GETTING HELP FOR OURSELVES

While working through what I can only describe as a soul crushing crisis, I had to develop ways to keep myself healthy, both physically and emotionally. Below are some suggestions that I have found to have a profound and positive effect on getting through this type of traumatic event.

You and I know what despair and hopelessness feels like. It is that dark place that we find ourselves in that keeps us from wanting to get out of bed in the morning. It is a sense of deep loss and sadness that overtakes us when we are looking at our loved one in the hospital bed with tubes and wires, and wonder if they will ever speak to us or even recognize us again. It is the darkness that envelops our minds and heart. We are in despair. We are grieving. And in order to make it through our grief, we must be willing to take a risk and share our sorrow with others who understand such grief and are safe and supportive. Whether it is your church, a support group, family or a trusted friend, go with what feels right for you and don't be afraid to reach out to others.

I remember the first time a friend of mine suggested that I attend a support group meeting. I was in denial, but she saw my inward pain and knew I needed help. In my mind I thought, "I am strong; I can handle this on my own". The truth be told, I was hurting on such a deep level and the sadness was something I just couldn't 'shake off'. I cried every night in private but couldn't understand why I was still so sad? My pain was not because of Orion's condition. In fact, he was improving. I thought, "Why are you hurting? He made it, and he's getting better. What's wrong with you?" The reality was that I had been traumatized and the pain was devastating. So one evening I decided to go to a meeting. After all, what could it hurt?

I sat in amazement while I listened to the people share their struggles and describe the healing process that occurred as they made their way through their own difficult circumstances. All of them were at different stages in their journeys. There were no judgments and no advice, just caring and supportive people allowing each other to 'get it out' and work their way through their own situation. They were compassionate people with listening ears and open hearts. I couldn't speak. I had never attended a place where people shared their innermost thoughts and feelings. I could feel the healing take place throughout the room as people shared their stories.

After the meeting, I was shocked to find myself running down the corridor to my car with tears pouring from my eyes. I was holding so much pain inside that it began to burst out of me and I had no clue how to make the hurt go away. A friend grabbed my hand and said, "It's okay". I quickly realized that I had been holding the entire trauma of Orion's accident inside and the emotions were pouring from my soul.

I went on to attend several more meetings, but it would be months before my mouth would open and the words would spill out. Then one day, out of nowhere, while sitting in the group, my story poured out like a flowing river. I had grown to trust these people and knew it was a safe place to share. Just as it had been with others who came before me, there were no judgments. Finally, I had let go and trusted the process so that *my* healing could begin.

Had I not listened to my inner voice and began attending meetings, I may have never met Barbara Whitfield at a convention the following year. I remember sitting in the room during the presentation as the speaker suggested we stand up, pick someone in the room and tell them something nice about themselves. I raised myself out of my chair and before I knew it, Barbara stood before me. We exchanged kind words as directed by the lecturer and took our seats. At the time I had no idea she would be the guest speaker later that day. It is *No Accident* that God brought us together or that we found ourselves at lunch later that day, discussing what you now hold in your hands. It's simply amazing how God works, when we listen and learn to trust the process.

It's important that we work through our grief or we may find ourselves becoming 'depressed'. Barbara's husband, Dr. Charles Whitfield, author of **Healing the Child Within**, calls this condition 'stuck grief'. (See his reference and contact information in the Resources section of this book.) He suggests that when we share our grief in a safe and supportive environment, we work through it and avoid those soul dampening feelings that accompany what we call 'depression'. The following is an excerpt from Fr. Whitfield's latest book. He is an expert in the field of Post Traumatic Stress Disorder (PTSD).

PTSD

Post-Traumatic Stress Disorder is not only for victims of TBI, war, rapes and car crashes. It also occurs in the families of those victims. It can occur when we have unresolved grief –from our losses. It can also occur in families where addictions, abuse, neglect and abandonment are present.

PTSD is an anxiety disorder that occurs when we or someone we know has had their life threatened –or they were harmed or killed. When long-term abuses, neglect abandonment occur to us, PTSD can form. When we are unable to grieve our losses, it can form. Dr. Charles Whitfield, a top specialist in the field describes PTSD, where it may arise and its manifestations (from his book, *Wisdom to Know the Difference*):

The Downside of Unresolved Grief

Emotional pain and PTSD: Unresolved grief festers like a deep wound covered by scar tissue, a pocket of vulnerability ever ready to break out anew. When we experience a loss or trauma, it stirs up energy within us that needs to be discharged. When we do not discharge this energy, we allow the stress to build up to a state of chronic distress. Trauma savvy clinicians and researchers call it PTSD. With no release this chronic distress is stored within us as discomfort or tension that may at first be so subtle that it is difficult for us to recognize it. We may feel or experience it through a wide range of manifestations such as **chronic fear, anxiety, tension** or **nervousness, anger** or **resentment, sadness, emptiness, lack of fulfillment, confusion, guilt, shame** or, as is common among many who grew up in a troubled family, as a feeling of numbness. These feelings usually come and go. There may also be **difficulty sleeping, aches, pains** and **other somatic complaints,** and **full-blown mental, emotional** or **physical illness**, including **PTSD**. In short, we pay a price when we are not allowed to and do not grieve in a complete and healthy way.

Though PTSD is not an easy-to-grasp problem, as its manifestations and causes may seem hidden to us, it is important and well worth our time to look into the possibility of PTSD if we have any of the manifestations listed above.

A trauma-savvy or PTSD-aware clinician can help.

Learn where to find more information on PTSD in the **Resources** section of this book.

A simple fact exists for you and me: we must work through our grief because we cannot avoid, minimize, alter or deny it. We can try, trust me I did, but it followed me like a freight train, fast on my heels. The only path to get beyond it is through it. To accomplish this, we need to call upon others who are experienced with the process. There are many successful groups to help us work through our pain and begin to heal.

Support groups offer tools and camaraderie. They are filled with safe and supportive people who will allow us to grieve in their presence, so that we can begin to move on with our lives. It is critical that we step out of isolation and ask for help. Procrastination only prolongs the inevitable. Eventually we need something or someone to guide us into the next phase of our journey. Remember, none of us are alone. All we have to do is take that first step.

There are several highly effective organizations in most towns and cities that have the kind of people, tools and atmosphere to help us work through our grieving process. Many references and contacts for these organizations can be found at the end of this book in the Resources section. Maybe for you it is a trusted friend, pastor, or a counselor; someone that you trust to talk to so you can "Get it out ". It's ok to cry. I didn't know the buckets of tears that would flow as I walked the path of healing. I also found solace in writing in a journal. It helped me to write about my innermost pain and emotions and then when I was finished I would burn the pages and would visualize the pain "burning away "as the paper evaporated into ash.

FINDING YOUR HIGHER POWER

I mention several times in this book that I hold a belief in a Higher Power, which I choose to call God. I know that many of us have prayed and have either not received the answers we wanted, or in some cases, the problems have worsened. We may have felt that whatever Higher Power was out there had abandoned us. I get that. I too said several times, "Why Him God, Why my son?" I felt abandoned by God in the beginning and had to work very hard to reconnect to my Source.

If you feel life challenges have become too big for you and you don't know where to turn, I understand. I too was desperately searching on the outside until one day I became still enough to hear the inner voice you hear when you learn to quiet your mind. It was inward that I found my strength to carry on.

In that connection to Source, at the heart level, we can experience stillness between ourselves and our Creator. It's through that stillness and connection to Source that I found my strength and my answers were revealed.

In my spiritual classes, I was taught that we are all a piece of God. I also learned to trust my Higher Power, which wasn't always easy as I was angry and felt cheated. At the time I felt as if my life had been ripped out from underneath me; that what had happened to my son was unfair. I had so many questions for God. Trust me; when I was in the trenches and desperately doing anything and everything to get my child back, anger, resentment, confusion, the whole gambit, drifted to the forefront of my mind. Let's face it; we need help during these times when it seems the universe has turned us into the butt of its worst and most oppressive joke.

Following my son's accident, I found out all too quickly that I did not possess the tools and stamina necessary to handle such grief and severe loss all alone. I began to feel the despair that I talked about earlier. In the end, I discovered that I needed something outside of myself that could actually be my solace and help me through this inhuman loss. I needed my connection to my Source, as well as my support group, family and friends. I didn't have to go it alone, and guess what, neither do you.

If you feel abandoned by whatever Higher Power you believe in, that is a legitimate beef. You have the right to that feeling, and don't believe anyone who tries to tell you that you don't. We are each on our own journey and life isn't always easy along the way. It's okay to ask a lot of questions. That's how we learn and grow. It is in asking and then listening, that we find the answers. However, in times of despair, we sometimes cannot hear the answers when they come. Our mind sometimes plays tricks on us. We are in a state of uncertainty and confusion and we need support.

Each of us chooses our particular beliefs. Your Higher Power may be associated with a specific religion or organization. For me, it is more about spirituality. I prefer not to put a label on my religion or religious beliefs. Rather, I am a spiritual woman and a piece of God and that feels right for me. My belief is spirituality is that part of us that transcends our physical nature. It connects us to each other with awe, trust, faith, compassion, love and other positive emotions. When I allow myself to connect spiritually to others and the universe, I stop feeling alone, unsure or separated.

I do not know from what source your Higher Power is derived, but I can share with you some that I have become acquainted with over the years. I know of individuals who have found solace in St Germain and the *I Am* teachings, which includes the use of the violet transmuting flame. Others prefer Native American practices surrounding the Great Spirit. There are those who find help in some forms of Christianity, Hindu, Dharma, or the teachings of the *Course in Miracles*. Some have found Buddhism fills their heart with practical meaning and compassion. They believe it helps one let go of his or her own ego, which they feel gets in the way of being their true self and causes them to suffer. I remember on a recent visit to see the Dali Lama, the compassion that I felt while in his presence. His radiance was so strong that I could feel it in the air as I sat at the end aisle with a clear opening and a bird's eye view. I imagined love and compassion going from my heart to his as I sat mesmerized by his presence.

Remember, your Higher Power must be what feels right for *you*. There is no right or wrong choice. Try to keep your mind open to a new experience. If the path you have chosen is not working, then by all means find another. Your sense of hope, wholeness and serenity may depend upon it. Whether you track an old, familiar path or experience a new one, my hope is that your connection to your Source helps you to accept and live life on life's terms, as well as find the serenity that you are hungry for.

NUTRITION AND EXERCISE

I found out early on that it was important to take care of myself. At times, removing myself from my loved ones, for any length of time, made me feel guilty or seemed impossible given all the responsibilities I had to fulfill each day. But if we don't take the time to fuel and exercise our bodies, we suffer the wrath of burnout, which is common amongst caregivers.

In the beginning, I couldn't seem to find the time, nor did I realize the importance of physical fitness, including regular consumption of healthy foods. However, as time went on I realized that when I didn't take time to care for myself, I had less energy and wasn't of service to myself or anyone else. I had to take time to focus on my own health, which included eating herbal foods as part of my daily regime. Visit **www.nourishnewbeginnings.com** for more information on the herbal foods I used to help myself stay well nourished.

Presently, I take time weekly to visit the local farmers market and try to get back to the life that I enjoyed before the accident. Eating healthy is a choice and I have learned to listen to my heart as well as my body. This is what 'feels' right to me, and I have learned to listen to that inner voice, even though my mind sometimes tries to convince me otherwise. I choose to listen and take the time for myself, it's a conscious decision. It's not always easy to make that choice as we may feel guilty. Please realize that there is no guilt in taking time to eat right and care for yourself. In fact, if you don't, burnout is likely and you will be of little service to anyone, including yourself.

It is just as important to take time for exercise, whether it is working out at a gym, walking, swimming or any activity that helps you work out some of the anxiety and physical tension that collects throughout the day. I personally take pleasure in outside scenery, rather than being stuck inside my house, trapped in my mind. As the saying goes, "The mind is a dangerous neighborhood to be in. Don't go there alone." Instead, I enjoy riding my bike around the block and long walks in nature. As I stroll along, I connect to my Source and allow any buildup of tension to soak into mother earth beneath my feet. The smell of her fresh air and the feel of her wind in my face rejuvenate me so that I can face whatever challenges the day may present.

Another activity that helps me is swimming. I have always been drawn to the water and that is where I find my peace. Swimming is a way for me to let my worries float away with the tide, while I envision all of my uncertainties drifting out to sea at the same time.

I also practice Kundalini yoga, which is a way of tuning into my spirit and my Source of life. Yoga helps calm my emotions and helps me to feel connected to life around me. As I let go and quiet my mind, I find a clear space that allows the healing to begin. I may be tense going into class, but when I leave I feel alive, refreshed and revitalized.

The extra stresses that you and I are under during this crises –on top of our normal life-- quickly depletes us of energy, We're in it for the long haul so, I can't stress enough how important it is to nurture your body, mind and spirit. My experience has been that as I better care for myself, I have more to give to the ones that I love.

Some friends remind me, "*Remember you can't give away what you don't have.*" So, I have to remember to take care of myself first so that I have the energy, strength and presence of mind to help others.

I would like to suggest that you try to exercise a little each day, even if you start with a simple walk around the block. It takes just a few minutes. It doesn't matter what activity that you choose or how much time you have available. Just allow yourself the time to heal and rejuvenate.

In the beginning I felt guilty leaving my son for even a minute, but soon realized that I was on the fast track to burnout and had to learn to take that time for myself. As I did, I had more energy to give my son and my loved ones.

Check out the YMCA, community centers, your local gym and your doctor for exercise options that are right for you. If you are a part of a TBI support group, you could ask what resources they may have available.

MEDITATION

I personally feel meditation is an essential part of my day. It is a time and space where I can shut off the world and connect to my Source, or "Higher Power." It wasn't always easy for me to halt the constant chatter in my mind, however now that I can quiet my mind and go inward; I find that space where I can hear God and where my answers are revealed.

You can connect to your Higher Power in a private meditation setting, or your connection can be as simple as communicating with your Source on a walk in nature. It doesn't matter what time of day or night it is. It doesn't matter whether the place you choose is a Sunday morning at church or a Friday night on a park bench. It's all your choice and there is no right or wrong way. It is what 'feels' right for you. Take the time to quiet your mind; even if it's only a few minutes a day. You will be happy that you did.

Many meditation and yoga centers offer *free* meditation instruction. Many centers have beautiful, quiet spaces that are conducive to meditation, and may provide a nice location to quiet your mind and relax naturally.

Perhaps searching the Internet for "Shambhala" centers, the local YMCA and community centers might turn up meditation instruction.

LIVING LIFE ON PURPOSE

My belief is that we are all a piece of God, connected to Source. And when we allow ourselves to tune into our Creator, we can feel the energy that is in our hearts. Have you ever heard a passage similar to 'all things I do, you too can do and more?' This is so true yet hard to imagine that we as human beings are capable of so much. I believe that as we choose to tap into that higher energy, the meaning of this passage strengthens. And its power becomes more apparent to me each time I watch the miracles unfold before my eyes.

Our thoughts are powerful. An example is when Orion chose to believe he could drive, rather than allowing his focus to remain on what others had said; that he could not and would not ever drive. It's no surprise that one of my son's favorite quotes developed early on in his recovery was, 'Whether you think you can or you think you can't, you're right.' You see, it works both ways. It's how we choose to view the outcome that makes the difference.

As I write my message, I sit and stare in amazement at all the beauty around me this very moment; the loudness and broadness of the ocean as the waves crash along the shore, the sparkling white light of the sun as it dances across the ocean and the coolness of the soft ocean breeze and the beauty of the palm trees as they sway in the breeze. In front of me is a lovely little sunflower that stares at me from a vase with three others that are wilted, yet I focus on the one that reaches for the sky. You may be wondering how I can allow myself to see, hear and feel such splendor when my loved one is struggling. It's sometimes not easy, but I've come to realize that as I changed my focus from what was *wrong* to what was *possible*, my world started changing too. I try to live by the words that God delivered to me through my son, to 'Never give up'. I truly believe that life is in divine order.

Now as I go through my days, I treasure the important things in life; My Higher Power, my family, friends and nature. I have always had a fulfilling relationship with God, but through this experience I have a renewed faith and trust in His guidance. The sound of my family's laughter, the time I share with friends, the beauty and smell of flowers, the coolness of a soft summer breeze, and the sound of the ocean crashing along the shore enlighten my life. When I rise each morning, I ask God, "How may I serve today, God?" Then I go about my business and experience His miracles as my day reveals itself. I choose to live my life on purpose, one moment at a time.

It's No Accident

My hope is that this book reaches a parent, grandparent, spouse, sibling, child or a patient with TBI or anyone who has given up hope. I pray that it finds itself in the hands of that person and sparks a flame to keep them going, so they may help their loved one or themselves move beyond all of the obstacles that seem to block each step along their path.

I realize that each and every brain injury is unique and each and every recovery is individual. I also know that no two outcomes are the same; however it is my belief that through love, faith, persistence and with God, all things *are* possible.

Yes, it takes hard work. Yes, doubt rears its ugly head. My mind drifts back to those long, dark days that seemed endless. I can still hear the sound of my son's whisper, "I'm here to teach you something, mom. Never give up!" I feel like the most blessed woman in the world. I have two brilliant sons. They are both independent and becoming the men that God intended them to be.

It is *No Accident* that the words found on that single piece of paper survived scattered amongst the hundreds of others destroyed within the wreckage of my son's car. Orion's journey was written by him, well in advance of the accident. I quote, "If our destiny is in fact predetermined then it must remain hidden in order to preserve the struggle. I too believe this to be an adventure in enlightenment." I believe that God has a plan for each and every one of us.

I thank you, my readers, for taking the time to read this book. I believe that it is *No Accident* that you did. It has been my pleasure to reach out with my heart, to share my experience, strength and faith, and offer you several tools to assist with the challenges that life places before you.

With all my heart and soul, I wish you strength, love, patience and wisdom, as you make your way through your own situation. May the light of God be with you and your families as you travel your own path to the truth!

> From my heart to yours,
> Carla Faith Christy

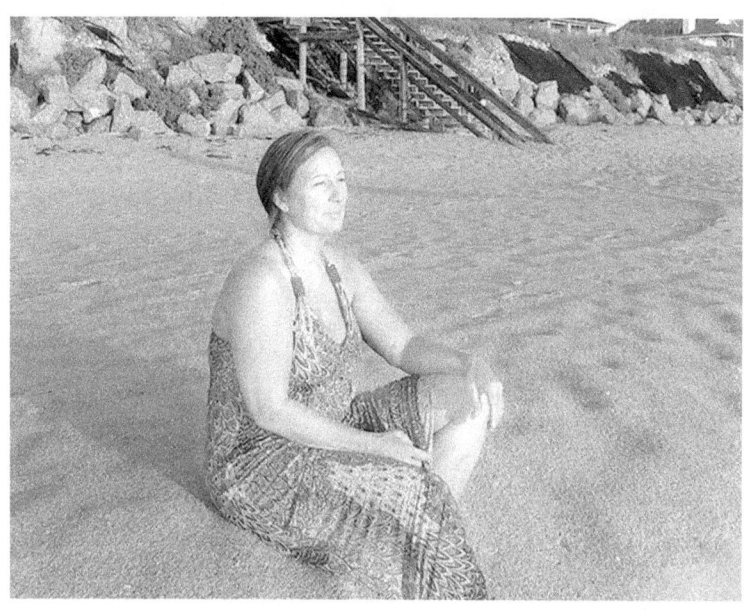

REFERENCES

Brooks, D. and Meinert L. (1998). Training Manual for Certified Brain Injury Specialists (CBIS) - Level I (2nd, Ed.). Alexandria, VA: American Academy for the Certification of Brain Injury Specialists.

Comparison of Annual TBI Incidence Chart at
www.biausa.org/Pages/pie_color.html

Daytona Beach News Journal

Resources

NoAccidentCarla.com
NoAccidentCarla@blogspot.com

For more information about Orion today, please visit his website at
www.orionchristy.com

Traumatic Brain Injury website at
www.TraumaticBrainInjury.com

Brain Injury - Pathogenesis, Monitoring, Recovery and Management, ISBN 978-953-51-0265-6
www.intechopen.com/books/show/title/brain-injury-pathogenesis-monitoring-recovery-and-management

Brain and Spinal Cord injury Program at
www.doh.state.fl.us/demo/brainsc/index.html

Brain Injury Association of Florida at
www.biaf.org

Herbal Food Info www.nourishnewbeginnings.com or email
Carla@nourishnewbeginnings.com

Brain Injury - Functional Aspects, Rehabilitation and Prevention, ISBN 978-953-51-0121-5
www.intechopen.com/books/show/title/brain-injury-functional-aspects-rehabilitation-and-prevention

ACA
www.AdultChildren.org

Alcoholics Anonymous
www.AA.org

Al-Anon Family Groups/Al-Anon for Adult Children/ALATeen
www.Al-Anon.org

Barbara and Charles Whitfield MD.
www.BarbaraWhitfield.com
Barbara-Whitfield.blogspot.com

Center for Grief & Healing
www.hns.org/Portals/1/Stages%20of%20Grief.pdf
From Center for Grief & Healing, Danvers, MA 01923, (978) 774-5100
www.griefandhealing.org

Co-Dependents Anonymous
www.CoDA.org
Living (or grew up) with any kind of Addict; alcoholic, drug addict, sex addict, religious addict, mentally ill, chronically ill, abusive or Codependent family member(s

National Institutes of Mental Health
www.NIMH.gov
Search on PTSD

Self-Realization Fellowship
www.yogananda-**srf**.org

Book Recommendations

1. Brown B (2010) On numbing our vulnerability. bipolarblast.wordpress.com/2011/11/06/we-numb-vulnerability/
2. Brown B (2010) *The Gifts of Imperfection*: Let go of who you think you're supposed to be and embrace who you are. Hazelden, Center City, MN
3. Brown N, Amatea E (2000) *Love and Intimate Relationships:* Journeys of the Heart. Philadelphia, Bruner-Mazel
4. Brown NM, Amatea ES (2000) *Love and Intimate Relationships:* Journeys of the Heart. Brunner/Mazel Philadelphia, Penn.
5. Campbell J (1949) *The Hero with a Thousand Faces*. Princeton University Press
6. Campbell J (2003) *The Hero's Journey:* Joseph Campbell on his life and work, 3rd edition, ed. Phil Cousineau. New World Library
7. Ekman P (ed.) (2008). *Emotional Awareness*: Overcoming the Obstacles to Psychological Balance and Compassion: A Conversation Between the Dalai Lama and Paul Ekman. New York: Henry Holt and Company
8. Griffin J. Clinical Depression (retrieved from www.clinical depression.co.uk/depression-article/ plus www.humangivens.com/joe-griffin/washington-times.html
9. Griffin J, Tyrrell I (2003) *Human Givens*: A new approach to emotional health and clear thinking. HG Publishing, UK
10. Griffin J, Tyrrell I (2007) *How to Master Anxiety*: All you need to know to overcome stress, panic attacks, phobias, trauma, obsessions and more. HG Publishing, UK
11. Johnson B (2005) *Emotional Health*: What emotions are and how they cause social and mental diseases. Trust Consent Publishing, Isle of White, UK
12. Katie B (2008) *Who Would You Be Without Your Story?* Hay House, NY
13. Klein M, Riviere J (1964) Love, guilt, and reparation in *Love, Hate, and Reparation*. Norton, NY, NY
14. Kurtz E, Ketcham K (1993) *The Spirituality of Imperfection*: Storytelling and the search for meaning. Bantam NY
15. Langer EJ (1975) *The Psychology of Control*. Sage, 1000 Oaks, Ca
16. L'Abate L (1977) Intimacy is sharing hurt feelings: A reply to David Mace. J Marital & Family Ther. 3:2, 13--16, April

17. Osbon DK (1991) *Reflections on the Art of Living*: A Joseph Campbell companion. HarperCollins, NY
18. Peck MS (1998) *People of the Lie*: The hope for healing human evil. 2nd ed. Touchstone
19. Papp LM, Cummings EM, Goeke-Morey MC (2009) For richer, for poorer: Money as a topic of marital conflict in the home. *Family Relations, 58,* 91-103
20. Simonov PV (1986) T*he Emotional Brain*: Physiology, Neuroanatomy, Psychology and Emotion. Springer, NY
21. Simos B (1979) *A Time to Grieve*: Loss As a Universal Human Experience. Families Intl, L.A. Ca
22. Stein W (1989) *On the Problem of Empathy*. In The Collected Works of Edith Stein, 3rd revised edition, ICS Publications, Washington DC
23. Welwood J (2000) *Toward a Psychology of Awakening.* Shambhala Publications, Boston, MA
24. Whitfield BH 2010 *The Natural Soul:* Unity with the Spiritual Energy that Connects Us. Muse House Press, Atlanta, GA
25. Whitfield CL (2010) Psychiatric drugs as agents of trauma. *Int J of Risk and Safety in Medicine* 22 (4)195-207
26. Whitfield CL (1987) *Healing the Child Within*: Discovery and recovery for adult children of dysfunctional families. Health Communications, Deerfield Beach, FL also *translated and published in* French, German, Spanish, Portuguese, Italian, Farsi, Japanese, Croatian and Korean translation editions
27. Whitfield CL (1990) *A Gift to Myself*: A personal workbook and guide to Healing the Child Within. Health Communications, Deerfield Beach, FL also *translated and published in* a French edition
28. Whitfield CL (1991) *Co-dependence* - Healing the Human Condition. The new paradigm for helping professionals and people in recovery. Health Communications, Deerfield Beach, FL 1991
29. Whitfield CL (1993) *Boundaries and Relationships*: Knowing, Protecting and Enjoying the Self. Health Communications, Deerfield Beach, FL - also *translated and published in* French and Spanish editions

30. Whitfield CL (1995) *Memory and Abuse*: Remembering and Healing the Effects of Trauma. Health Communications, Deerfield Beach, FL
31. Whitfield CL, Silberg J, Fink P (eds.) (2002) *Misinformation Concerning Child Sexual Abuse and Adult Survivors*. Haworth Press NY
32. Whitfield CL (2003) *The Truth about Depression*: Choices for Healing. Health Communications, Deerfield Beach, FL, (800-851-9100) (translated into Portuguese) Two chapters published in Goldberg R (2006) *Taking Sides*: Clashing Views in Drugs & Society (7th Ed) McGraw-Hill, Dubuque, IA)]
33. Whitfield CL: *The Truth about Mental Illness*: Choices for Healing. Health Communications, Deerfield Beach, FL, 2004
34. Whitfield CL (2003) *My Recovery: A Personal Plan for Healing.* Health Communications, Deerfield Beach, FL
35. Whitfield CL, Whitfield BH, Prevatt J, Park R (2006) *The Power of Humility*: Choosing Peace over Conflict in Relationships. Health Communications, Deerfield Beach, FL
36. Whitfield CL (2010) *Choosing God:* A Bird's Eye View of A Course in Miracles. Muse House Press, Atlanta, GA
37. Whitfield CL (2010) *Teachers of God*: Further Reflections on A Course in Miracles. Muse House Press, Atlanta, GA
38. Whitfield CL (2011) *Not Crazy:* You May Not Be Mentally Ill - Misdiagnosed and mistreated with drugs that don't work well or make you worse. *Important information withheld from you by the Drug Industry, Psychiatry, Government, and others.* Muse House Press, Atlanta, GA
39. Whitfield CL (1984) *Alcoholism, Other Drug Problems & Spirituality*: Stress Management and Serenity During Recovery. Perrin & Tregett, Rutherford, NJ
40. Whitfield CL (2006) The Doctor's Opinion. in *Adult Children: Alcoholic/Dysfunctional Families.* [the first "Big Book" of Adult Children of Alcoholics] Torrance, Ca/Brainerd, MN
41. Whitfield CL, Whitfield BH (in process for 2013) *Engaging the Muse*: Using Creativity in Everyday Life. Muse House Press, Atlanta, GA
42. Jill Bolte Taylor PHD (2006) My stroke of insight, penguin group (USA) Ny,NY

More from Muse House Press

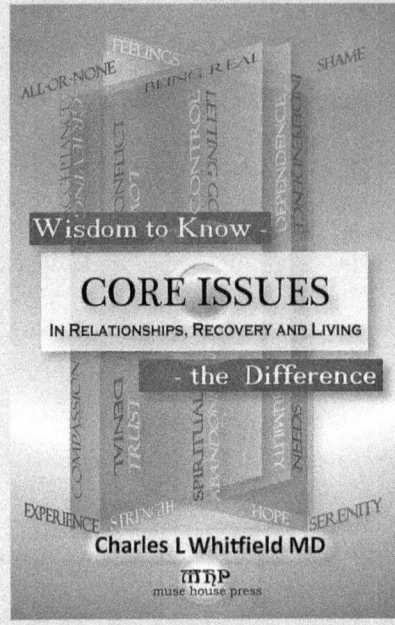

This book addresses in detail these common Core Issues in Relationships Recovery and Living.
» Needing to be in control
» Difficulty trusting
» Difficulty being real
» How to handle feelings
» Low self-esteem (shame)
» Dependence & Independence
» Fear of abandonment
» All-or-non thinking
» High Tolerance for Inappropriate Behavior
» Over-responsibility for others
» Neglecting my own needs
» Grieving my ungrieved losses
» Difficulty resolving conflict
» Difficulty giving/receiving love

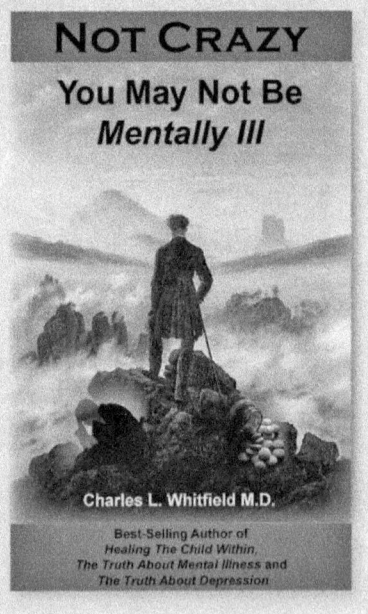

"In my over 30 years assisting countless people with a variety of mental, emotional, behavior, and relationship problems, I have come to realize that many of them have been misdiagnose and mistreated. In fact, most o them were not mentally ill. In this book I share research and experience and offer hope and another way that may success-fully address what may not be a "mental illness"

—Charles Whitfield MD

Other Helpful Books By The Whitfields

Dr. Whitfield takes us into the heart and soul of *A Course in Miracles*.

This book is an <u>excellent</u> companion to reading the Course itself.

—Jyoti & Russell Park, PhD
Center for Sacred Studies, California

co-authors of
The Power of Humility
Choosing Peace over Conflict in Relationships

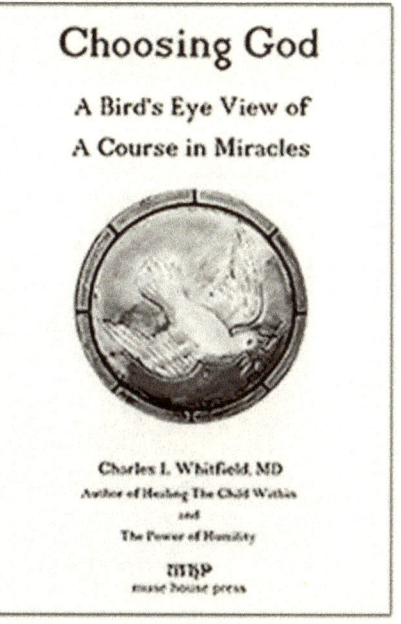

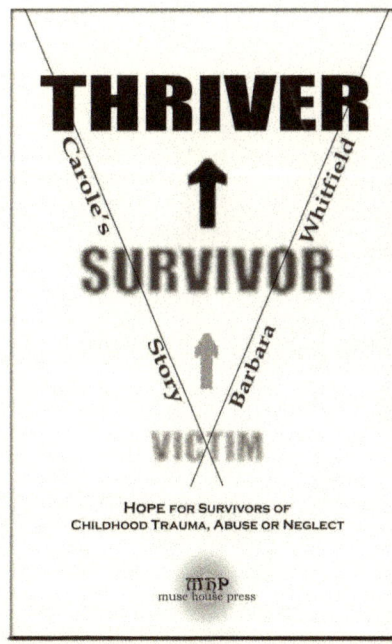

This is not an easy book to read. It contains real-life pain, sadness and loss. Some of us have suffered like Carole did --and worse-- yet in reading this book – we discover healing. There is help here. And most importantly, there is hope within these pages for anyone who has been severely and repeatedly traumatized, abused and/or neglected in childhood. Whitfield quotes from Carole's documentary: "The thunderstorms are just as beautiful as a sunny day. And so is life!"

—Donald Brennan
Certified Addiction Counselor
from the Foreword

More from Muse House Press

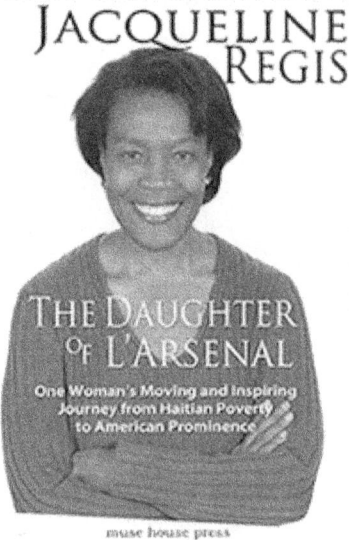

A inspiring story of a woman of two worlds. In this moving memoir of love and driven determination against all odds, Jacqueline Regis, an accomplished lawyer and judge, tells the story of her climb up from poverty in Haiti to prominence in America in vivid and stirring detail. She shares with us the hope and inspiration to keep reaching higher for our goals, and never giving in to anything less.

This book will inspire you to make the most of your life!

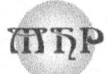

"...many tools and techniques to help the reader transform the ordinary difficulties of life into moments of calm, clarity and, sometimes, surprisingly, even the deepest joy. And they do it not only skillfully but with humor, too. This is a book to treasure --and to keep handy."

Kenneth Ring, PhD
Author of
Lessons from the Light

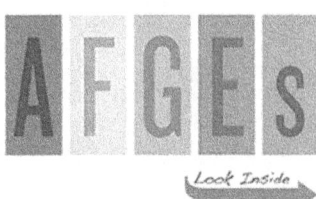

A Guide to Self-Awareness and Change

BARBARA HARRIS WHITFIELD AND SHARON K. CORMIER
Foreword by Charles L. Whitfield, MD

www.ingramcontent.com/pod-product-compliance
Lightning Source LLC
Chambersburg PA
CBHW032357040426
42451CB00006B/42